Coping Successfully with Psoriasis

CHRISTINE CRAGGS-HINTON

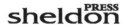

First published in Great Britain in 2008

Sheldon Press
36 Causton Street
London SW1P 4ST

The author and publisher have made every effort to ensure that the
external website and email addresses included in this book are correct and
up to date at the time of going to press. The author and publisher are not
responsible for the content, quality or continuing accessibility of the sites.

British Library Cataloguing-in-Publication Data
A catalogue record for this book is available from the British Library

ISBN 978-1-84709-047-8

1 3 5 7 9 10 8 6 4 2

Typeset by Fakenham Photosetting Ltd, Fakenham, Norfolk
Printed in Great Britain by Ashford Colour Press

Produced on paper from sustainable forests

Cc

Christine Craggs-Hinton, mother of three, followed a career in the civil service until, in 1991, she developed fibromyalgia, a chronic pain condi-

t

ן

L
t
new
too.

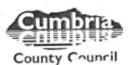
Cumbria
County Council

Libraries, b

Overcoming Common Problems Series

Selected titles

A full list of titles is available from Sheldon Press,
36 Causton Street, London SW1P 4ST and on our website at
www.sheldonpress.co.uk

Body Language: What you need to know
David Cohen

The Chronic Pain Diet Book
Neville Shone

The Complete Carer's Guide
Bridget McCall

The Confidence Book
Gordon Lamont

Coping Successfully with Varicose Veins
Christine Craggs-Hinton

Coping with Age-related Memory Loss
Dr Tom Smith

Coping with Compulsive Eating
Ruth Searle

Coping with Diabetes in Childhood and Adolescence
Dr Philippa Kaye

Coping with Diverticulitis
Peter Cartwright

Coping with Family Stress
Dr Peter Cheevers

Coping with Hay Fever
Christine Craggs-Hinton

Coping with Hearing Loss
Christine Craggs-Hinton

Coping with Kidney Disease
Dr Tom Smith

Coping with Polycystic Ovary Syndrome
Christine Craggs-Hinton

Coping with Radiotherapy
Dr Terry Priestman

Coping with Tinnitus
Christine Craggs-Hinton

Depression: Healing Emotional Distress
Linda Hurcombe

Every Woman's Guide to Digestive Health
Jill Eckersley

The Fertility Handbook
Dr Philippa Kaye

Free Yourself from Depression
Colin and Margaret Sutherland

Helping Children Cope with Grief
Rosemary Wells

How to Be a Healthy Weight
Philippa Pigache

How to Get the Best from Your Doctor
Dr Tom Smith

The IBS Healing Plan
Theresa Cheung

Living with Birthmarks and Blemishes
Gordon Lamont

Living with Eczema
Jill Eckersley

Living with Schizophrenia
Dr Neel Burton and Dr Phil Davison

Living with a Seriously Ill Child
Dr Jan Aldridge

The Multiple Sclerosis Diet Book
Tessa Buckley

Overcoming Anorexia
Professor J. Hubert Lacey, Christine Craggs-Hinton and Kate Robinson

Overcoming Emotional Abuse
Susan Elliot-Wright

Overcoming Hurt
Dr Windy Dryden

Overcoming Insomnia
Susan Elliot-Wright

Overcoming Shyness and Social Anxiety
Ruth Searle

Reducing Your Risk of Cancer
Dr Terry Priestman

Stammering: Advice for all ages
Renée Byrne and Louise Wright

Stress-related Illness
Dr Tim Cantopher

Tranquillizers and Antidepressants: When to start them, how to stop
Professor Malcolm Lader

The Traveller's Good Health Guide
Dr Ted Lankester

Treating Arthritis: More drug-free ways
Margaret Hills

Contents

Note to the reader   vi

Introduction   vii

1   Psoriasis   1

2   Plaque psoriasis   9

3   Other forms of psoriasis   18

4   The cause of psoriasis   43

5   Creams and lotions   49

6   Pills and injections   61

7   Phototherapy   75

8   Self-help   80

9   Psoriasis and nutrition   92

10 Emotional help   103

11 Complementary therapies   116

Useful addresses   129

References   132

Further reading   133

Index   135

Note to the reader

This is not a medical book and is not intended to replace advice from your doctor. Consult your pharmacist or doctor if you believe you have any of the symptoms described, and if you think you might need medical help.

Introduction

Psoriasis – a complex skin disease – is difficult to live with on both physical and emotional levels. The condition is now known to be genetic, lying dormant for a lifetime in many cases. For others, however, it is triggered into action by such things as smoking, drinking too much alcohol, stress or injury.

Having skin that is repeatedly violated by red scaly patches is far from easy. Women and younger people seem to experience the most distress – women because they tend to be very image conscious and younger people because they hate being different in any way from their peers, particularly if they're in their teenage years and it's in a way that makes them feel less physically attractive than other people of their age. That's not to say men aren't affected by the way psoriasis makes them look – they certainly are, but usually not to quite the same extent.

Contrary to public opinion, the condition doesn't only present cosmetic concerns. Getting on with everyday life can be a real problem too, for the areas affected can itch unbearably and it can make you feel out of sorts. People with severe psoriasis – particularly if it is psoriatic arthritis, or plaque psoriasis that has caused splits in the skin of their hands – often find that their dexterity is affected and may have difficulty even with punching numbers into a telephone, brushing their teeth and signing their names. Thankfully, in a physical sense, very few are so badly affected. However, the majority are affected in an emotional sense and may even fall victim to chronic anxiety or dark depression.

Psoriasis brings a myriad of conflicting emotions. For instance, the fact that there is, as yet, no cure for the condition and that flare-ups keep on recurring is usually a source of great anger, frustration and despair. Frustration also comes from the sense of being unable to control what's happening to you and your body, which is perhaps the most difficult aspect of all.

Although over two per cent of the population have psoriasis, few people understand what it's all about. It's only when you receive a diagnosis that there are suddenly a million questions, yet doctors are often too short of time to answer them all. That's where a book such as this comes in.

Most people with psoriasis feel that their quality of life is negatively affected. They feel they are being judged on their appearance, and they may respond by covering themselves in long sleeves and long trousers or by staying indoors and away from staring eyes. This book aims to teach coping strategies that boost confidence and self-esteem, allowing you to get more out of your life.

In the following chapters I discuss the different forms of psoriasis together with the causes of the condition, the triggers and various types of self-help, including a good healthy diet that can only be of benefit. The book also contains a number of treatment strategies, ranging from creams and ointments to pills and injections and finally phototherapy (the use of light as a treatment). I hope very much that the chapter offering emotional help is of real value, too. Finally, there is a chapter discussing the complementary therapies believed to be useful in treating psoriasis.

1

Psoriasis

Psoriasis – pronounced with a silent *p* – is a common skin condition that affects at least two per cent of the population. The disorder is classed as chronic, meaning long-lasting, and it generally occurs in 'bouts' that consist of a rapid-onset flare-up of variable length followed at some point by a healing period, also of variable length. Most people learn to recognize the early signs of a flare-up.

Until a few years ago, experts believed that psoriasis was the result of an immune system fault that caused the rapid multiplication of skin cells in certain areas. However, recent research has shown us that in as many as a third of cases, the cause is genetic – i.e. people with particular genetic differences have a weakened immune system and are more susceptible to developing the condition. Psoriasis lies dormant until triggered into action by factors such as stress, smoking, certain weather conditions, alcohol consumption, infection or injury.

A person with patches of the rough, scaly skin characteristic of psoriasis may experience a great deal of cosmetic embarrassment and distress. There are also physical symptoms that vary in severity, for even mild psoriasis can cause itching, burning, stinging and a general feeling of being unwell. Psoriasis is graded as mild, moderate or severe, depending upon how much of the body is affected.

In some people, the symptoms of this condition can be so incapacitating that it is impossible to live a normal life, and the gradual outcome is depression and social isolation. The physical and emotional aspects of psoriasis can even increase the risk of alcohol abuse and of consuming too many non-prescription drugs. Many people with psoriasis smoke or drink caffeine in an effort to reduce the emotional impact of the condition, but these forms of self-medication only make things worse, for psoriasis reacts adversely to all such substances.

Psoriasis does not only affect the skin – indeed, the fingernails, toenails and joints can be attacked. When the nails are affected, they become discoloured and thickened, and when the joints are affected it causes them to become inflamed (psoriatic arthritis), the result of which can be mild, moderate or severe disability. The only life-threatening forms of psoriasis are the widespread types such as erythrodermic psoriasis and generalized pustular psoriasis, but it is only in very rare cases that they are severe enough to endanger life. In erythrodermic psoriasis a red peeling rash usually covers the whole body, and in pustular psoriasis there are many tiny red bumps that are filled with non-infectious pus.

As plaque psoriasis accounts for up to 90 per cent of psoriasis cases, this form of the condition is discussed in detail in Chapter 2. The other types of psoriasis are examined in greater detail in Chapter 3.

The history of psoriasis

Psoriasis has plagued humanity for many centuries – it is even mentioned in a set of 2000-year-old Greek medical chronicles. For hundreds of years it was believed to be a kind of leprosy, which made it a condition to be greatly feared and avoided at all cost. Sadly, the leprosy taint was still evident in the late eighteenth century, when English dermatologists Robert Willan and Thomas Bateman distinguished it from other skin diseases and gave it the name 'Willan's lepra'. The leprosy link wasn't lost until 1941, when Viennese dermatologist Ferdinand von Hebra re-named the condition 'psoriasis' (taken from the Greek *psora*, which means to itch).

Psoriasis was not subdivided into its different forms until the twentieth century. (See Chapter 3 for information on the different forms of psoriasis.)

Who gets psoriasis?

Although most experts are of the opinion that psoriasis affects males and females equally, a few studies have indicated that it may be more common in men than in women. The condition is not generally associated with type of employment, although butchers and people who come into contact with animal skins have been found, for some reason, to stand a greater chance of developing the condition. There is also statistical evidence that there are a slightly higher number of homes in which both partners have psoriasis than homes in which only one partner has the condition. Experts believe that this is due largely to the fact that, when they first meet, people with psoriasis find they share a common bond and so want to become better acquainted.

Although psoriasis can arise at any age, an estimated one in ten of the psoriasis population develops the condition during childhood (see page 6 for more information about children with psoriasis). In rare cases the condition can occur in infants or, at the other end of the scale, it may first arise during your 50s or 60s. However, the signs and symptoms of psoriasis most commonly appear between 15 and 35 years of age. When the condition starts early in life it is referred to as type I psoriasis, and when it starts later in life it is known as type II psoriasis.

Interestingly, some studies have discovered that psoriasis develops in colder climates at an earlier age, and that it is more widespread in such places. For example, the condition is more prevalent in African-Americans and white-skinned (Caucasian) people who live in colder climates than in people of any racial group who live in the hot climates of Africa. The condition is also more prevalent in the colder climates of Scandinavia and other parts of northern Europe.

As mentioned, psoriasis is a genetic condition. Research has indicated that when both parents have psoriasis, their children appear to have a 50–75 per cent chance of developing the condition, whereas if only one parent is affected, the children appear to have a 25 per cent chance of developing it. The possible genetic component is explored in greater detail in Chapter 4.

Can you get only one type of psoriasis?

Psoriasis may begin in one form but then develop later into another form entirely. For example, plaque psoriasis can change into guttate or erythrodermic psoriasis, the latter two of which are described in

Chapter 3. Abruptly stopping a psoriasis medication such as methotrexate or ciclosporin can bring this about.

In addition, two forms of psoriasis can co-exist at the same time. For example, when plaque psoriasis is already present, a second type can appear, such as pustules developing around the plaques. In this situation, the person has plaque psoriasis and pustular psoriasis. (Pustular psoriasis is discussed in Chapter 3.)

It is possible to experience one outbreak of psoriasis in isolation. This is most likely to occur with guttate psoriasis, as discussed in Chapter 3. In rare cases, one solitary flare-up can occur with other forms of psoriasis, too.

Is there a cure for psoriasis?

Although there is currently no cure for psoriasis, the genes responsible for causing the condition have now been identified and scientists hope that at some point in the future they will be able to modify them safely. In the meantime, experts envisage that more effective treatments and therapies for the various forms of psoriasis may be developed.

Is psoriasis catching?

Psoriasis is not catching or transmissible in any form or at any stage of its existence. It can't be transferred from one part of the body to another, and it can't be passed to other people – if it could be, many doctors would have it! If you are in any doubt about this, ask your doctor for reassurance.

Is there a link with skin cancer?

Some people think that the increased rate of cell division in psoriasis means there is a greater risk of skin cancer. Unfortunately, there is some evidence that people with severe psoriasis who take any type of drug that affects the whole body (systemic medications) are at greater risk of developing primary skin cancers and lymphomas, but the risk is only very slight. In patients with mild and moderate psoriasis, the risk is thought to be no higher than normal.

Is psoriasis caused by a 'state of mind'?

There is still a tendency to think that rashes of any kind are caused by 'nerves' – i.e. by the way you are feeling. Indeed, after diagnosing psoriasis, doctors are repeatedly asked, 'Is it my nerves, do you think?' Doctors used to believe that the skin largely acted as a reflection of the person's innermost self, producing a rash at times of stress and a skin disease at times of great anxiety and nerviness. It's true that at such times some people become blotchy and maybe develop pinprick spots, but these normally disappear when the thing that caused the stress or embarrassment is over. Otherwise there is no link between skin diseases and the way you are feeling. Once you do have a skin disease, however, it can be made dramatically worse by your state of mind.

The gravity of psoriasis

Psoriasis varies immensely in gravity. For some people it is no more than a mild nuisance, whereas for others it can be disabling – particularly when linked with arthritis (see Chapter 3). Widespread psoriasis – particularly pustular psoriasis and erythrodermic psoriasis – can even be life-threatening in rare cases.

There are now grades for the gravity of psoriasis, based on:

- the percentage of the body affected;
- the degree of disease activity (for instance, in plaque psoriasis, the amount of redness, scaling and thickness would be assessed);
- the reaction to any previous medications; and
- the effect of the disease on the individual person, such as the degree of stress or depression caused.

Here are the grades:

- Psoriasis is classed as *mild* when it affects less than five per cent of the body's surface.
- It is classed as *moderate* when it affects 5–20 per cent of the body's surface. Many experts assert that the cut-off point should be lowered to 10 per cent, particularly when taking into account cases that affect the hands or feet.

- It is classed as *severe* when it affects more than 20 per cent of the body's surface.

It has been estimated that approximately 67 per cent of people with psoriasis are mildly affected, 25 per cent are moderately affected and 8 per cent are severely affected.

Resistant areas

Unfortunately, any form of psoriasis in the following areas can be resistant to treatment:

- on the palms of the hands and soles of the feet
- in the folds of the skin
- on the scalp.

Psoriatic arthritis can also be difficult to treat.

Children with psoriasis

In children, it seems that the earlier psoriasis shows itself, the more likely it is to be widespread and recurrent. The appearance of plaque psoriasis (see Chapter 2) in adults is slightly different from its appearance in children – the lesions are not as thick and scaly. In infants with psoriasis, the plaques often occur in the nappy area, as well as in skin creases and in areas where two surfaces of skin are in contact – under the arms, beneath the buttocks and so on. In children, psoriasis commonly arises on the scalp before spreading to other areas. It is also likely to form on the face and ears, which it rarely does in adults.

The effect of pregnancy on psoriasis

Psoriasis does not endanger pregnancy in any way. Indeed, a recent survey indicated that pregnancy can actually generate an improvement in symptoms. The survey in question followed 47 women with psoriasis during the course of their pregnancy, comparing them with 27 non-pregnant women with psoriasis. An improvement in symptoms was reported by over half of the pregnant women – however, within six weeks of giving birth, most experienced a worsening of symptoms. Interestingly, there was a significant improvement in symptoms during the tenth to twentieth week of pregnancy, when oestrogen levels are beginning to peak, and it is this rise in oestrogen levels that is believed to be responsible for the improvement.

Of far more concern than the effects of psoriasis on pregnancy are the effects of medications available to treat psoriasis – when given to a pregnant woman they are liable to cause miscarriage or severe birth abnormalities that can lead to the child's death (see Chapter 6). Therefore, if you are planning to get pregnant, it is vital that you seek your doctor's advice, particularly if you use medications to control your psoriasis.

Phototherapy (treatment with light) is a far safer option than medications, but afterwards plenty of moisturizers need to be used to prevent plaques from drying out too much. Severe cases of psoriasis can be treated by topical cortisone cream, but its application should be limited to problem areas rather than used to cover large body surfaces – cortisone cream is a corticosteroid and it can be absorbed into the body and cause problems for the developing child.

If you have psoriatic arthritis and wish to get pregnant, you should be aware that the condition can be particularly problematic during this time. Fortunately, many arthritis medications can safely be used during pregnancy. Speak to your doctor if you have psoriatic arthritis and are planning a pregnancy.

Psoriasis and skin colour

The dysfunctions evident in psoriasis are the same in all persons regardless of the colour of their skin. However, there are believed to be variations in the genetic susceptibility for developing the condition between people from different areas of the world. For instance, the prevalence of psoriasis is much lower in dark-skinned West Africans and African-Americans than in light-skinned northern Europeans.

The emotional impact of psoriasis

Having a skin condition – whether it is widespread or restricted to one or two visible areas – can knock your confidence and make you want to shrink away from other people. Women are possibly more self-conscious and therefore more prone to depression and social isolation than men, though this is not always the case. See Chapter 10 for advice on dealing with the emotional impact of psoriasis.

When to see your doctor

You should see your doctor if you are not comfortable with how your skin looks and feels. The presence of raised red patches with silvery scales is a clear give-away – particularly if there is more than one and they have appeared within a few days after an injury to the skin, however slight the injury was. Less obvious symptoms include red patches on the skin, which may itch, or dry areas of skin, which may be scaly and peeling.

If you are in any doubt at all, go to your doctor.

2

Plaque psoriasis

Although the correct medical term for the most common form of psoriasis is plaque psoriasis, the word 'plaque' is usually dropped and the condition is referred to simply as 'psoriasis'.

Skin cell overgrowth and inflammation are present in all forms of psoriasis, but in plaque psoriasis there are recurrent 'flare-ups' of patches (known as 'plaques'), which are either a bright red colour or a dull red wine colour. These patches, or plaques, are slightly raised and may vividly stand out from the normal skin colour. Moreover, they are often covered in silvery scales and can itch immensely, which in itself is distressing. The unsightly red patches are also a cosmetic concern, causing distress and loss of confidence.

The plaques

Plaque psoriasis begins with the development of a small red bump on the skin that may be pinprick size or up to 3 mm (about an eighth of an inch) in diameter, with a circular or oval shape. Any other patches in the area may give a rash-like appearance – however, the patches soon begin to spread out and merge, taking on an irregular outline where several patches have joined up and formed a larger area.

As the patches grow larger, they feel dry and rough to the touch, becoming more shiny and silver as dry scales form. In some people, the patches become ring-shaped, with a definite centre and raised scaly borders. The patches can grow so large that they eventually cover wide areas of the chest or back – these are known as geographic plaques because they resemble maps. Any injury to the plaque such as a scratch or scrape causes spots of blood the size of pinheads.

The number of scales can depend on the location of the particular patch, how long it has been present and the type of treatment, if any, that it has received. For example, patches in sensitive areas such as under the breasts in a woman are usually without scales; the longer a patch has been present usually makes for more scales, and taking particular systemic drugs has the potential to clear the patch as well as the scales. (See Chapters 5, 6 and 7 for information on psoriasis treatments.) The main areas that tend to have scales in large numbers are the arms, legs, trunk and scalp.

Unfortunately, there is currently no cure for any form of psoriasis. For some people, plaque psoriasis completely clears for years at a time, occasionally never returning at all. In most cases, however, it is a life-long condition with alternating bouts of flaring and clearing. Significant relief can be achieved, however, with the aid of modern medicine – usually on a permanent basis – together with the use of self-care techniques. The medications and self-help techniques are described in this book.

How much does psoriasis hurt?

In plaque psoriasis, there is a wide spectrum of possible sensations. Most people experience a degree of discomfort or soreness, whereas a smaller percentage of people have to contend with itchiness, stinging and a burning sensation (this can be very distressing) – and some lie somewhere in between.

Trying to lift off the scales with a fingernail will cause bleeding, and the area can bleed when unintentionally injured, such as from an injection, being rubbed by tight clothing, being knocked against a chair, or being burned (e.g. from being brushed against a hot iron). A vicious circle can then develop, for yielding to the itching can provoke a flare-up – and when a flare-up is in progress, further plaques will usually arise in any part of the body, particularly in places where a minor injury might occur during the flare-up.

When a plaque is so dry that it begins to crack and bleed, the resultant pain may be so sharp and intense that it can be difficult to concentrate, and even sleeping may be a problem. If infection sets in, there may also be a certain amount of discomfort, even pain, and as the affected area begins to heal it will start to itch, whether or not it has itched before.

The location of the plaques

Plaques can form on any part of the body – even, in rare cases, the eyelids, ears, mouth, lips, palms of the hands and soles of the feet. However, the knees, elbows and lower back are the most common sites. Plaques can also arise in the genital areas in both men and women, as well as above the pelvic bone and on the thighs and calves.

In some cases, the patches occur symmetrically, in the same position on either side of the body. In about 50 per cent of cases, the plaques spread to the scalp, sometimes becoming thickened and

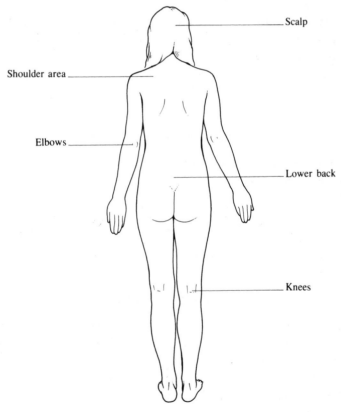

Figure 1 Areas of the body most affected by common forms of psoriasis

occasionally extending down to the forehead. They seldom appear on the face, however, especially in adulthood.

Places on the body most affected by common forms of psoriasis are shown in Figure 1.

Plaques on the scalp can cause a lot of discomfort and often cosmetic concern. For most, there are only a few small scaly areas, but for others, the scalp becomes covered in crusty patches that are hard to conceal, and these patches can cause snowstorms of white flakes that look like dandruff – an embarrassing problem. Scalp psoriasis is discussed in Chapter 3.

Not all psoriasis patches are topped with silvery scales. In regions where two skin surfaces are in close contact – i.e. in natural skin creases and folds such as beneath a woman's breasts, under the buttocks, beneath the arms and in the groin and genital area – psoriasis plaques remain raised and red, and they can also appear shinier than psoriasis plaques in other areas. These areas may be enormously itchy and can burn, but for plenty of people they cause no discomfort at all.

The unique features of psoriasis

Certain other skin conditions are similar in appearance to psoriasis. However, psoriasis has some unique features:

- Psoriatic lesions have clearly defined edges.
- On the surface of the lesions there are usually silvery scales that easily flake off.
- Beneath the scales the skin is shiny and red.

How skin works

Healthy skin has the important role of regulating body temperature, keeping in the body's fluids and acting as a protective barrier against injury and infection. However, when the skin is affected by a disease such as psoriasis, changes occur that alter its behaviour and ultimately undermine its efficiency.

Normal skin cells

When normal skin is viewed under a microscope, it is evident that there are two main parts:

- The *dermis* is the strong, elastic inner layer of the skin. It is composed of tendons, ligaments and nerves, as well as the tiny blood vessels – called capillaries – that provide the skin with oxygen and nourishment. The dermis is also composed of tough fibres called collagen, which gives healthy skin its flexibility and pliancy.
- The *epidermis* is the thinner outer, visible layer of the skin. The epidermis is composed of several layers of cells that are produced at the base and move up to the surface, changing shape and structure as they become filled with a fibrous protein called keratin. When they eventually reach the top layer they drop off. This whole process is known as keratinization.

The structure of normal skin is illustrated in Figure 2.

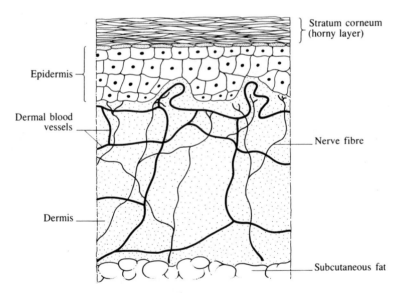

Figure 2 Structure of normal skin

The disease process in psoriasis

The disease process begins in the bottom layer of the epidermis where immature skin cells (called keratinocytes) that produce the tough protein called keratin are formed. It normally takes about a month for keratinocytes to multiply and travel from the lower layer of the skin to the surface, unobtrusively shedding cells as they go. However, in psoriasis, they multiply and travel to the surface in only four days, and because the cells cannot be shed quickly enough, they accumulate in thick dry patches, which are the plaques characteristic of plaque psoriasis.

Because the process is speeded up, many more cells than normal lie within the epidermis. As a result, the epidermis takes on a more folded appearance than usual (see Figure 3) – however, the folding is only visible through a microscope. Among this overabundance of cells are blood vessels, which are also trapped in the folding

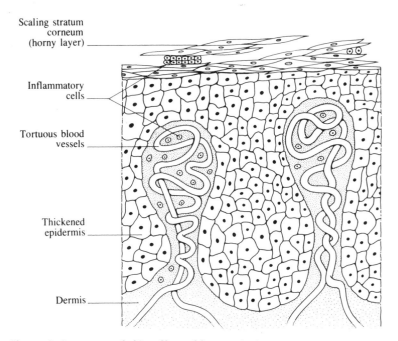

Figure 3 Structure of skin affected by psoriasis

epidermis. Such vessels become much wider, too, and the blood they contain flows more quickly than normal, increasing the blood supply to the skin. This explains why psoriasis patches are red and bleed easily.

The underlying skin – the dermis – accommodates nerves, blood vessels and drainage channels (called lymphatic vessels). Together these provide the blood supply and drainage for the abnormally multiplying keratinocytes. This blood supply also transports white blood cells, which create the underlying inflammation and contribute to the redness.

Some of the white blood cells increase inflammation by straying into the outer layer of the skin (epidermis). These white blood cells can gather together and form small abscesses or pus spots, as seen in pustular psoriasis.

Abnormal skin function in psoriasis

When psoriasis occurs, the skin becomes far less effective at keeping out infections, including bacterial infections, toxins and other harmful substances. The skin of someone with psoriasis also allows fluid from the tissues to seep out and evaporate more quickly than normal into the air around them – up to ten times as fast in some cases. This is of little consequence when only a small area of skin is affected, but the fluid loss can be substantial in people with severe, widespread psoriasis. Mild dehydration may even occur, showing itself as a dry skin and tongue, or a greater thirst than normal.

A further consequence of plaque development is that the skin becomes weaker and more rigid than it was, sometimes cracking in areas that are put under strain, such as on the hands or around the joints. Cracks in such areas can be painful and a cause of great deal of aggravation. They can even make it difficult to function.

The fact that the skin in psoriasis is likely to allow substances to enter more easily than normal can be turned to advantage, for creams and ointments are absorbed very well. This surprising outcome presents us with an easy way of effectively treating the condition in many cases. Topical treatments such as creams and ointments are discussed in Chapter 5.

Psoriasis and body temperature

As mentioned earlier, the skin plays an important role in regulating body temperature. However, it has been seen that in psoriasis, the temperature regulatory system is often disrupted. Indeed, the temperature of a person with widespread psoriasis before treatment is likely to be lower than normal. Fortunately, it has been observed that after treatment, body temperature reverts to normal.

Low body temperature can occur due to blood flow in a patch of psoriasis being faster than average, which makes the skin feel and look unusually warm. However, the person may actually be cold and shivery, particularly if there are multiple patches of psoriasis on the body. Widespread psoriasis can even cause such a drop in body temperature that mild hypothermia occurs. It makes sense then to say that spending a long time outdoors on a freezing cold day could possibly encourage hypothermia for people with psoriasis, and that that keeping warm is the best course of action.

Because psoriasis scales can potentially block a pore through which perspiration comes out – our bodies use perspiration as a means of cooling down – it is also possible to become hotter than normal. If you have widespread psoriasis and are spending time in a hot climate or kitchen, or have a raised temperature due to an illness such as influenza, your temperature may start climbing to alarming heights – a condition known as hyperthermia. Your best course of action here is to remove most of your clothing and lie down with a cold flannel on your forehead. Applying ice packs should help, as should placing a fan close by. It's also important that your doctor sees you.

How psoriasis differs from other skin conditions

Having an area of red, scaly skin doesn't automatically signify psoriasis. There are a few other skin conditions with a similar appearance, the main one being eczema, or dermatitis. Psoriasis and eczema are often confused with each other. However, each requires completely different medication. Sometimes even doctors get it wrong and diagnose eczema when the problem is psoriasis, and vice versa.

The difference between psoriasis and eczema

The main difference between psoriasis and eczema is that the borders of psoriasis patches are clearly defined, unlike those in eczema. Eczema is usually itchier than psoriasis, but not always. Indeed, very itchy psoriasis plaques are a prime reason that doctors can misdiagnose the condition.

The difference between psoriasis and ringworm

Ringworm – caused by a fungal infection – can also resemble psoriasis. The difference is that ringworm patches usually occur in isolation, unlike psoriasis. Ringworm, as the name suggests, occurs in ring shapes.

Does psoriasis go away?

Doctors find it difficult to forecast the behaviour of psoriasis in a particular patient, for it can follow a wide variety of courses. In some people, there are small inconspicuous patches of plaque psoriasis behind the knees or elbows that remain unchanged throughout that person's lifetime, whereas for others, similar small patches can seem to expand suddenly until they cover large areas of the body. Conversely, widespread plaque psoriasis with large patches that crack and become infected can unexpectedly start to calm down and fade – maybe even disappearing from view – without any treatment. It would seem, then, that psoriasis can indeed go away. Don't be fooled, however. It goes into remission, that's all. The condition almost always comes back at some point.

Medical professionals have found that psoriasis is usually 'mild and persistent'. In other words, the disease is a minor nuisance for many years – periodically getting worse when numerous patches emerge, followed by times of vast improvement, when the skin appears quite normal. Fortunately, times of flare-up are usually short-lived, while periods of improvement can occur over long stretches of time.

Although the other forms of psoriasis are rare, they are generally more of a problem than plaque psoriasis. The other forms are discussed in Chapter 3.

3

Other forms of psoriasis

Of the various forms of psoriasis, some exist in isolation whereas others occur at the same time as other variants. It is not unknown for one form of psoriasis to disappear, to be followed by another.

Areas of the body affected by the less common forms of psoriasis are shown in Figure 4.

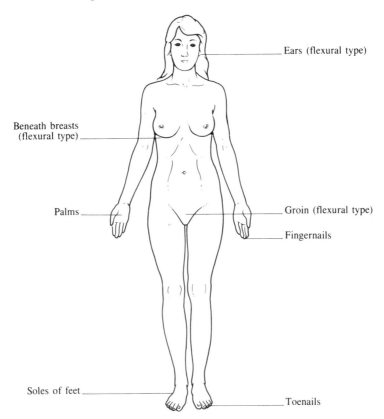

Figure 4   Areas of the body affected by less common forms of psoriasis

Treatment of psoriasis depends largely upon the type of psoriasis, where it is, how severe it is, and the person's age and overall health. How much the person is physically and emotionally affected by the condition is also taken into account.

Plaque psoriasis, the most common variant, was discussed in Chapter 2; this chapter is devoted to helping you to understand the remaining forms.

Psoriatic arthritis

Arthritis is often wrongly considered to be a medical condition in itself when in fact it is the label for a group of over 100 disorders in which inflammation is present in the joints and sometimes in muscles, tendons, ligaments or bones. One of this group is psoriatic arthritis (sometimes referred to as PsA, for short), which can occur in 7–15 per cent of the psoriasis population and which usually starts between the ages of 30 and 50. As with other forms of psoriasis, white-skinned people (Caucasians) are more likely to develop the condition than people of other races.

Psoriatic arthritis is a relapsing–remitting disease characterized by inflammation in the joints, particularly the joints of the fingers and toes, which causes them to be swollen and painful. The majority of people with this form of arthritis also have the patches of dry, scaly skin that are typical of plaque psoriasis, and a massive 80 per cent have a condition known as nail psoriasis, which is described later in this chapter. It is common for people with psoriatic arthritis to suffer from inflammatory eye conditions such as conjunctivitis.

Although flare-ups of psoriatic arthritis are liable to take place at the same time as those of plaque psoriasis, experts are not yet certain whether it is a unique disease or a form of psoriasis. However, recent evidence suggests that they are both caused by the same immune system dysfunction.

A famous person with severe psoriatic arthritis was Dennis Potter, arguably the most important creative figure in the history of British television. Potter turned to writing after the onset of psoriatic arthritis, producing dozens of TV scripts, books and plays. His work always managed to reflect his real-life struggles with psoriasis and psoriatic arthritis. He even managed to be productive when his hands became crippled, strapping a pen to his hand to continue writing. Another notable person with psoriasis was the American novelist John Updike – and there was also the abominable Adolf Hitler.

There is currently no cure for psoriatic arthritis, but in most cases it is not nearly so debilitating as other forms of arthritis. Medical treatment is essential, however, together with physiotherapy and, if applicable, beneficial lifestyle changes such as giving up smoking and drinking and getting more exercise. In cases where the condition is not tackled by treatment of any kind, there may be persistent discomfort and progressive joint damage, leading eventually to disability and deformity.

Faulty immune system function makes people who are infected with human immunodeficiency virus (HIV) more likely to have psoriatic arthritis than those who are HIV-negative. Existing psoriasis may also be worsened by HIV infection.

Making the diagnosis

In psoriatic arthritis, problems with the skin and joints don't usually develop at the same time, yet doctors look for both problems when attempting to make a diagnosis. Most people have skin symptoms long before problems in the joints occur – maybe even decades before; however, a relatively small number of people experience joint inflammation and pain before skin symptoms emerge. There is even a very small number who don't ever have skin symptoms. My brother has psoriatic arthritis, yet he has never been troubled by skin problems. Therefore, it was many years before doctors were able to make a diagnosis.

A diagnosis of psoriatic arthritis can also be hampered by the presence of skin symptoms at the same time as any condition that causes pain in the joints, such as osteoarthritis, rheumatoid arthritis, gout or Reiter's syndrome. Very mild skin problems can delay a correct diagnosis, too.

As no single test can confirm a diagnosis of psoriatic arthritis, doctors generally look for:

- pain, redness, swelling and reduced motion in the joints, especially the small joints at the ends of the fingers and toes; although uncommon, there may also be similar symptoms in the joints of the spine and sacroiliac (the two large joints that connect the pelvis with the triangular bone at the end of the spine);

- fatigue and stiffness in the morning;
- pitted, discoloured nails that may be coming away from the nail beds;
- a susceptibility to inflammatory eye conditions such as conjunctivitis.

A systemic disease

As you can see from the list of diagnostic pointers above, psoriatic arthritis is a *systemic* disease – that is, it affects the whole body, whereas plaque psoriasis affects only the skin.

Types of psoriatic arthritis

Experts have defined five categories of psoriatic arthritis according to the problem areas and severity of joint involvement:

Symmetric psoriatic arthritis

Symmetric psoriatic arthritis occurs at the same place on both sides of the body and usually affects four or more pairs of joints. In approximately 50 per cent of cases the condition progresses, affecting more and more pairs of joints. Although symmetric psoriatic arthritis is similar to rheumatoid arthritis, it is usually much milder. However, its progression can still lead to disabling joint damage. More women than men are affected by this form of psoriatic arthritis, and the co-existing plaque psoriasis is often severe.

Asymmetric psoriatic arthritis

Asymmetric psoriatic arthritis is the mildest form of psoriatic arthritis. It is characterized by periodic pain and redness, usually in one to three joints on one side of the body or in different joints on each side of the body, causing them to be red, swollen and tender. The knee, hip, ankle, wrist and one or more fingers are commonly affected. When this type of psoriatic arthritis is present in the hands and feet, inflammation can cause a lot of swelling, making the fingers and toes resemble small sausages.

Distal interphalangeal predominant psoriatic arthritis

Distal interphalangeal predominant (DIP) psoriatic arthritis occurs in only about five per cent of psoriatic arthritis cases, mostly in men. It involves the joints of the fingers and toes, in the area closest to the nail. This variant of psoriatic arthritis is similar to osteo-arthritis, in which the bones become brittle and the cartilage wears away. However, osteoporosis does not cause nail problems, whereas DIP psoriatic arthritis does.

Psoriatic spondylitis

Psoriatic spondylitis describes inflammation of the joints of the backbone (spondylitis) – the chief symptom in about five per cent of psoriatic arthritis cases. Spondylitis related to psoriatic arthritis gives rise to stiffness and burning sensations in the neck, the lower back, the sacroiliac area (the joint between the sacrum at the base of the spine and the ilium in the pelvis) or the spinal vertebrae (the backbone), making movement difficult. Inflammation may also be present in areas where tendons and ligaments attach to the spine. There is thought to be some spinal (backbone) involvement in up to 75 per cent of psoriatic arthritis cases, although it is not generally the primary problem.

People with psoriatic spondylitis are at greater risk of developing osteoporosis. This causes the bones to become brittle, so that eventually even a minor stress like coughing can cause a fracture. It is advisable to get plenty of exercise and include a lot of calcium and vitamin D in your diet. If bone density scans carried out at intervals show that the slow destruction of your bones is continuing, you are likely to be prescribed drugs that slow down bone loss.

Arthritis mutilans

Arthritis mutilans is the most severe type of psoriatic arthritis, affecting less than five per cent of people with psoriatic arthritis. It is unfortunately very painful and deforming, and gradually worsens over time. The small joints of the hands and feet are mainly affected – indeed, the small bones in the fingers can slowly be destroyed, leading to deformity and disability. According to studies, bone destruction and deformity occurs in 5–16 per cent of psoriatic arthritis patients. Arthritis mutilans often attacks the neck and lower back, too. Flare-ups of arthritis mutilans and psoriatic skin problems usually occur at the same time.

Diagnostic tests

The following medical tests can help to distinguish psoriatic arthritis from other similar conditions:

- X-rays – changes in the joints peculiar to psoriatic arthritis can usually be seen on X-ray.
- Erythrocyte sedimentation rate – this blood test determines whether inflammation is present. As several conditions can cause inflammation in the body, this test cannot be solely relied on to make a diagnosis.
- Joint fluid test – in this test, a small sample of fluid is taken from one of the joints for laboratory analysis. The absence of uric acid crystals usually rules out gout, which is one of the conditions sometimes confused with psoriatic arthritis.
- Rheumatoid factor – this blood test indicates whether an antibody that is present in the body of someone with rheumatoid arthritis is in evidence. If not, rheumatoid arthritis can usually be ruled out.
- Other blood tests – haemoglobin levels may be checked because many people with psoriatic arthritis are anaemic.

The cause of psoriatic arthritis

Like all other forms of psoriasis, psoriatic arthritis is an autoimmune problem. This basically means that the body's immune system mistakenly attacks healthy tissue instead of doing its normal job of fighting harmful organisms such as viruses and bacteria. It is this abnormal immune response that gives rise to inflammation in the joints as well as the overproduction of skin cells – the root cause of the skin problems in psoriasis.

It is believed that both environmental and genetic factors play a role in causing the immune system to turn on itself, as happens in psoriatic arthritis.

A familial link

As psoriatic arthritis is believed to be a form of psoriasis and researchers have now identified a genetic component to the disease (see page 45), psoriatic arthritis is probably also genetic – in other words the predisposition towards having it probably runs in the family. Studies have found that almost half of the people with psoriatic arthritis have a close family member such as a parent or sibling with the disease. You don't automatically develop the disease if a family member already has it, but you will be susceptible to developing it if you experience a certain trigger, as discussed below. If you have psoriatic arthritis and there is no sign of any form of psoriasis in your family, it is likely that none of your family members have encountered a trigger.

Triggers

As explained above, psoriatic arthritis appears to remain dormant in the body until triggered by a specific occurrence of some kind, including the following:

- an infection, particularly of a streptococcal bacterium
- an injury to the skin, such as a burn, cut or scrape
- stress
- excessive alcohol intake
- poor nutrition
- reaction to a medication or vaccine
- overexposure to the sun or prolonged exposure to irritants such as disinfectants or paint thinners.

Children with psoriatic arthritis

A small number of children develop psoriatic arthritis, usually at around the age of nine or ten. The disease is mild in the vast majority, but in a few it can cause severe symptoms and disability that persists into adulthood. Most children display the same symptoms as adults, but there is a higher likelihood of skin and joint problems. As the bones are still forming in children, normal skeletal development can also be impaired.

Treatment

Medications

In treating psoriatic arthritis, the objective is to prevent further damage to the joints, reduce joint swelling and pain and improve any patches of dry, scaly skin. In order to achieve this, a combination of medications may be prescribed. Mild psoriatic arthritis can usually be treated by the use of non-steroidal anti-inflammatory drugs (NSAIDs) such as ibuprofen and aspirin to help relieve the morning stiffness, the inflammation and any pain. As NSAIDs can lead to gastrointestinal problems, they should only be used to control psoriatic arthritis symptoms on a short-term basis.

When NSAIDs are not able to relieve your pain and inflammation, other drugs may be prescribed:

- Cyclo-oxygenase-2 (COX-2) inhibitors – these drugs are similar to NSAIDs in that they reduce swelling, morning stiffness and pain, but because they are believed to be less irritating to the stomach, they are more likely to be tolerated. COX-2 inhibitors have been associated with a raised risk of heart attack and stroke, however.
- Disease-modifying anti-rheumatic drugs (DMARDs) – the aim of this type of drug is to prevent further damage to the joints. As DMARDs work slowly, it may be weeks or months before any benefit is felt. In the meantime, your doctor may prescribe a painkiller.
- Sulfasalazine – this drug was originally developed to treat inflammatory bowel disease, but it is now also extensively used to treat the symptoms of psoriatic arthritis. The possible side effects include nausea, vomiting and appetite loss, which can be relieved by the prescription of enteric-coated tablets (ask your doctor about this), or by lowering the dosage.
- Methotrexate – this drug can be taken by mouth or given by injection. It can reduce the symptoms of skin psoriasis and it can also reduce joint inflammation and damage, and even slow down the disease progression in some people. In low doses, this drug is well tolerated, but serious side effects, including liver damage, can arise when it is taken for long periods. (See Chapter 6 for more information about methotrexate.)

- Azathioprine – this drug was originally used to prevent organ rejection after transplants, but it is now used in severe cases of psoriatic arthritis. However, long-term use can increase the risk of malignant (cancerous) or benign growths occurring, as well as certain blood disorders. Nausea, vomiting, fatigue and easy bruising are other side effects.

Surgery

When other treatments fail to control symptoms, surgery may be recommended – although this is so only rarely. Various surgical procedures are now available, the aim of which are to relieve pain and restore mobility. As operations always carry a risk, discuss the matter thoroughly with your doctor and try to be sure that you choose the right option.

The outcome of surgery is largely dependent on the strength of the bones and ligaments that support the joints. Ability to take part in a rehabilitation programme also plays a part in the end result.

Self-help

Coping successfully with psoriatic arthritis also depends largely on self-help measures. For instance, cutting out cigarettes and alcohol, eating a healthy diet, maintaining a healthy weight, taking regular exercise, taking care of your skin, using relaxation techniques and pacing yourself can make a great difference. Self-help measures are discussed mainly in Chapter 8.

Nail psoriasis

Plaque psoriasis is frequently accompanied by nail psoriasis. Indeed, the two conditions so often exist side by side that when nail psoriasis occurs in isolation doctors can find it very difficult to diagnose. Having a family history of psoriasis can help in the diagnosis; however, nail psoriasis doesn't always run in the family.

Abnormal changes in the nails often appear before any other form of psoriasis. Indeed, studies have indicated that nail changes are present in about 86 per cent of people with psoriatic arthritis and in around 50 per cent of people with skin psoriasis.

The nail unit is composed of many parts, including the nail plate, nail bed, nail matrix, nail folds, cuticle, the anchoring part of the nail bed and the top part of the finger or toe bone (these bones are called the distal phalanges). In nail psoriasis, any of these areas can be affected, and obviously the problem can cause significant dysfunction – we use our hands and nails in numerous daily tasks, which can be made very difficult, or impossible, by problems with the nails. Moreover, the unsightly appearance of nail psoriasis can cause psychological distress, especially if the fingernails rather than toenails are involved. However, the appearance of psoriatic toenails can result in self-consciousness in summer, when open-toed shoes and sandals are worn, or during an outing to the beach or swimming baths.

Signs and symptoms

Here are the possible changes that point to nail psoriasis:

- There may be unusual nail discoloration – this is often of a translucent yellow–red tone in the bed of the nail, and it tends to look like a drop of oil or blood under the nail plate. Doctors often refer to this as an 'oil drop' or 'salmon patch'.
- There may be tiny white pits dispersed in groups across the nail, and each one may be shallow or deep. The pits occur when cells are lost from the surface of the nail. There may also be yellowish spots.
- There may be ridges across the nails, usually but not always going from side to side rather than up and down. They are actually growth arrest lines caused by intermittent inflammation.
- There is usually thickening of the skin beneath the nail, a condition called onychomycosis. This can lead to the nail becoming loose (see below).
- The nail can become loosened, a white area appearing where it is separated from its underlying attachment to the nail bed. The separation usually starts at the tip of the nail, extending down toward the root. Dead skin is likely to accumulate beneath the nail and the nail bed may become infected.
- Crumbling of the nail may occur. The nail can weaken, owing to the underlying tissue and cells being unhealthy.

- There may be deformity in the shape of the nail. As well as being caused by the immune system dysfunction that underlies psoriasis, this arises as a result of weakening of the underlying tissues.
- Tiny black lines running from tip to base may appear. This is caused by the capillaries bleeding at the tip of the finger or toe between the nail and the skin beneath the nail.
- The nail cuticle may appear red, owing to congestion of the capillaries beneath the nail.
- Arthritis in the fingers or toes may arise in people with nail psoriasis.
- Fungal infections of the nail can also occur in people with nail psoriasis, as can inflammation of the skin around the edges of the nail.

When to see your doctor

You should see your doctor if there are any unusual changes in your nails – for example, if they become discoloured, if pits appear, or if they are painful or seem to be infected. When you go to your doctor, he or she may take a small sample (biopsy) of the skin beneath your nail to determine the cause of your problems.

Treatment

Currently, there is no cure for psoriasis of the nails, but in some cases it improves by itself. The aim of any medical treatment is to improve your ability to function and to make your nails look better. If a fungal infection is present, an antifungal medication will be prescribed.

There are several drugs, ointments, creams and other therapies available for treating nail psoriasis, but they tend to be more effective when used in conjunction with general psoriasis medication, as well as with the self-help measures described in this book. When used alone they may prove disappointing.

The following treatments and self-help strategies may be suggested by your doctor:

- corticosteroid creams and lotions and corticosteroid-impregnated tape (for more information on these three treatments, see Chapter 5) and 5-fluorouracil;

- intra-lesional corticosteroid injections into the affected nail;
- phototherapy applied as 'paint' or taken orally (for more information on phototherapy, see Chapter 7);
- removal (by surgical means or application of a strong urea compound) of any nails that have been deformed by psoriasis;
- other repairs, such as the regular scraping and filing of nails that have become long and thickened.

You can also obtain advice on concealing nail discoloration with nail polish and on buffing and polishing to help to disguise pitted nails. In some cases, you may also be advised about the possibility of using artificial fingernails.

For people with severe, widespread psoriasis, the treatments being given for other areas of the body will determine their nail treatment. For example, methotrexate is often prescribed as a systemic treatment (treatments that affect the whole body, not just the skin), and it benefits the nails as well as the skin in psoriasis. Other psoriasis treatments such as phototherapy are of benefit to the nails, too. However, some systemic treatments are either of no help to the nails, or can actually make them worse. For instance, acitretin, which is used to improve psoriatic lesions, can cause the nails to become thin and abnormal in appearance. Fortunately, acitretin is usually prescribed as a short-term treatment to alleviate a flare-up, and when it is discontinued the nail changes resolve.

When nail psoriasis is accompanied by onychomycosis – a fungal infection of the nails that causes abnormal thickening – the doctor will usually prescribe a systemic antifungal medication. It is estimated that one-third of people with nail psoriasis struggle with fungal infections.

Ointments to remove the nail

If a nail is beyond repair and needs to be removed, your doctor will probably prescribe a urea-based tincture such as benzoin, with which you should thickly cover the nail, placing adhesive tape around it. In turn, this should be covered by a layer of cling film and adhesive tape to secure it in place. The mixture should be left on the nail for five to ten days, after which time the nail should come off cleanly, without any bleeding.

If the nail has been removed to deal with an infection, medication to treat the infection will continue to be prescribed.

Surgery to remove the nail

If other treatments fail, a doctor can use a minimally invasive procedure to remove the nail. A local anaesthetic injection will first be administered to ensure there is very little discomfort, then the nail will be removed at the base with an instrument called a needlepoint scalpel. Aftercare is similar to that of any minor surgical procedure, and the risks associated with surgical nail removal are minimal.

Caring for your nails

In most cases, it is possible to improve the condition of your nails by observing the following self-care advice:

- Keep your nails trimmed back to the point of firm attachment – this allows medications to be more effective. Longer nails are prone to rub against surfaces, and such trauma may trigger a flare-up of psoriasis or worsen an existing flare-up.
- Keep your nails as dry as possible. Don't wear shoes that may let in the rain and possibly trigger a psoriasis flare-up.
- Wear gloves while working with your hands.
- Try to avoid injury to the nails. Accidentally bumping and scraping the nails can provoke either a flare-up of nail psoriasis or a nail infection.
- Take great care when using implements for cleaning beneath the nails. Avoid vigorous scraping under the nail and over-enthusiastic cleaning. This may break the skin where the nail is attached.
- Psoriatic toenails will benefit greatly from soaking the feet for ten minutes daily in a bowl of warm water.
- If the toenail is thickened, carry out the following procedure while your foot is in the water: gently file the thickened area with an emery board, then, using clippers, cut off a tiny area of the thickened toenail at a time. Try to cut straight across the toenail to prevent it from becoming ingrown.
- Avoid wearing tight shoes if your toenails are thickened. There

should be room enough for the toes to move. The friction caused when walking in tight shoes can make toenails thicken.

Artificial nails

When psoriatic nails are damaged but basically intact, many people choose to improve their appearance by wearing artificial nails. It must be said, though, that artificial nails have been reported to worsen psoriasis in some cases and expose the wearer to infection and allergic risks. For instance, it is possible to have an adverse reaction to one or more of the chemicals used in the adhesive. A manicurist may be unwilling to apply artificial nails to nails that have crumbled or become deformed. However, numerous people are willing to accept the risk, particularly those with psychological distress related to their nails, and a large number experience no adverse reaction at all.

Scalp psoriasis

At least half of all people with plaque psoriasis have it on their scalp – indeed, some have it solely in this area. Scalp psoriasis is often very mild, appearing like a bad case of dandruff. However, in some people there are thick crusted plaques covering the entire scalp, extending beyond the hairline on to the forehead, around the ears and down the back of the neck. Such severe scalp psoriasis can be distressing because of the physical symptoms it causes, such as soreness, itching and a feeling of tightness, and because of the adverse psychological impact of its appearance. In addition, the appearance factor can be even more problematic because hair loss may also occur, though not by any means in all cases.

There are a variety of topical creams, lotions, gels and solutions to treat scalp psoriasis, but in severe and persistent cases systemic medications are often prescribed – in other words, instead of creams and so on that treat only the skin you are given a medication that enters the entire body and all the body systems. Such treatment is usually taken by mouth or received by injection. Topical products, on the other hand, are applied to the skin and, in most cases, are specifically designed to treat the skin.

Provided they seek medical help and use the recommended treatments, few people experience extensive scalp psoriasis over a prolonged period. Scalp treatments generally involve massage of a medication into the hair and scalp and must be repeated until adequate control is obtained. This may take eight weeks or longer. Once an acceptable clearing of lesions has been achieved, the use of a tar shampoo or other medicated shampoo (see below) twice daily can successfully keep the condition at bay. It may also be of benefit to moisturize the scalp regularly.

Hair loss

In cases of severe scalp psoriasis, there may be some temporary thinning of the hair. Obviously, this can be very distressing, particularly if your hair is thin anyway. Fortunately, the hair starts to thicken again once the flare-up is over. In the meantime, a man can best cope by wearing a hat or shaving his head bald. Investing in a wig for temporary use may be the best option for a woman who is very distressed about thinning hair.

Brushing and combing

If you are worried about brushing or combing your hair during a flare-up, there is no need to be, providing that you take care to avoid scratching your scalp. In fact, it is important that you do regularly comb or brush, since this can remove loose scales. Avoid being too vigorous.

Cosmetic hair treatments

Most cosmetic hairdressing procedures are safe for people with scalp psoriasis. However, it is best to have your hair styled and treated during a remission, when the disease is inactive. If there are scratches or open sores on your head, the chemicals in most treatments will cause soreness and irritation.

If you want to colour or perm your hair, rather than using a home kit you would be well advised to have it treated by a hairdresser who will have up-to-date information about the best options for people with psoriasis. Most of us tend to feel better when our hair has been styled or treated in some way.

Don't be embarrassed about going to a hairdresser. If you are worried about what the stylist will think of your condition, it is probably a good idea to telephone in advance to explain the situation. If you are worried about other customers, there are now many 'mobile' stylists who will visit you in your home.

Scalp psoriasis versus seborrhoeic dermatitis

A few other skin disorders resemble scalp psoriasis, but seborrhoeic dermatitis is by far the closest in appearance. In scalp psoriasis the scales seem powdery and have a silvery sheen, while the scales in seborrhoeic dermatitis appear yellow and greasy. In seborrhoeic dermatitis, there is also far less redness and no raised red areas. Severe seborrhoeic dermatitis appears as thick oily crusts and is most common and long-lasting in fair-skinned people.

Seborrhoeic dermatitis is often evident as cradle cap in infants, in whom it occurs as thick oily crusts. The infant form usually clears up by itself and does not predispose a person to the condition later in life. However, adult seborrhoeic dermatitis is a chronic condition that can evolve into psoriasis.

The two conditions are still easily confused, but fortunately their treatments are very similar.

Treatment

Tar

Occasionally, scalp psoriasis will clear on its own. When it doesn't, there are several treatments available, including tar products such as tar shampoos, creams, gels, oils, ointments, solutions and soaps – these can usually be purchased over the counter (without the need for a doctor's prescription) in a variety of strengths. Tar products can also be prescribed by your doctor. To use the shampoo, massage it into the scalp and leave for about five minutes before rinsing off. To decrease the smell of tar and to make the hair more manageable, use a conditioner, too. For a more intense treatment, tar gels, creams, solutions and lotions can be massaged into the scalp and left overnight. Tar treatments may also be used in combination with other forms of treatment.

Topical corticosteroids

Corticosteroids can also be of benefit for scalp psoriasis, particularly those that have been developed to treat the scalp. They come in solution, gel, cream, lotion, spray, foam and ointment form. Water- and alcohol-based preparations are easier to wash out of the hair after treatment.

Topical corticosteroids are available only on prescription, and they range from mild to very strong. Use them for no longer than two weeks, slowly reducing the application. Avoid using corticosteroid preparations near the face, eyes and other sensitive areas unless instructed to do so by your doctor.

A useful topical corticosteroid for the scalp is clobetasol propionate (brand name Etrivex). Clobetasol propionate is a strong topical corticosteroid known for its good success rate for clearing psoriasis.

Some topical treatments for scalp psoriasis don't work for some people, in which case another treatment such as betamethasone valerate (brand name Bettamousse) should be tried. If the skin on the scalp has become resistant to a treatment, it can take a few months for another treatment to work.

Intralesional corticosteroid scalp injections

In cases where psoriasis is mild on the scalp, corticosteroid medications can be injected into the lesions. As the medication can be absorbed into the body, a doctor will not inject into more than three or four areas.

Anthralin

Some people with scalp psoriasis respond better to anthralin, an older medication. When washed into the scalp, it must be left for only ten minutes before being washed off. A variation of this medication can be used in higher concentrations for a shorter period of time – it is known as short contact anthralin therapy (SCAT).

Because anthralin can stain the skin and possibly cause irritation, it is best applied in the shower and removed by being pushed to the back of the head before being washed off, directing the spray toward the back of your head. It is best to hold a face cloth over your forehead and eyes while rinsing the front of your hair. If you get the medication in your eyes, try to wash it out immediately, using an eyebath and solution such as Optrex. You may need to repeat the washing out process many times, and if the irritation continues, go to the accident and emergency department at your local hospital.

Antimicrobial therapy

In cases where the skin becomes infected, psoriasis of the scalp can worsen. If your lymph nodes enlarge or crusting of the scalp intensifies, an antimicrobial treatment may be prescribed. Antifungal shampoos such as Nizoral may also be of benefit. Such shampoos help to decrease the numbers of yeast organisms and so calm down the infection. They should be used once or twice a week until the infection disappears.

Medicated shampoos

Scalp lesions can be treated by coal tar and non-coal tar medicated shampoos. Follow the instructions as to how long the shampoo should be left before being washed out. Medicated shampoos treat the scalp, not the hair, and for this reason you may wish to use ordinary shampoo and conditioner as well. This may also make your hair more manageable and help to remove the smell of the medicated shampoo.

Guttate psoriasis

Guttate psoriasis is an unusual presentation of psoriasis. It is characterized by small, red, teardrop-shaped bumps which appear on the skin – the Latin word for 'drop' is *gutta*. This fairly uncommon type of psoriasis can look like a 'shower' of spots on the skin. It usually arises on the arms, legs and middle of the body (trunk), sometimes spreading to the face, ears or scalp. People of any age can have guttate psoriasis, but it is normally seen in older children and young adults under the age of 30. The condition is not contagious.

The 'drops' – which are sometimes referred to as lesions – may be covered with scales that are much finer than those seen in plaque psoriasis. They often present no more than a mild or moderate inconvenience, but sometimes they can itch. Their presence can also present a cosmetic problem, for they are not pleasant to look at and, if you have them, you may be inclined to hide your body. Guttate psoriasis drops on the face, ears and even the scalp are a more difficult problem, for they are not so easy to hide.

The condition usually comes on quite suddenly over a few days and is associated with a preceding cold or other infection – usually a streptococcal infection of the throat. Indeed, in a study of 62 patients with guttate psoriasis, it was seen that the condition was preceded by a clinical infection in 84 per cent of cases.[1]

Factors that can trigger guttate psoriasis include:

- a streptococcal infection (see below);
- upper respiratory infections – usually the common cold;
- tonsillitis;
- viral infections such as chickenpox, rubella (German measles) and roseola – all of these conditions are most common in children, the last-named being a fever and rash of sudden onset that can occur in children under two years of age;
- bacterial infections, such as those which occur when harmful micro-organisms enter a wound;
- injury to the skin, such as cuts, burns, insect bites and sunburn;
- stress;
- binge drinking or other alcohol abuse;
- some medications, such as some used to treat malaria and high blood pressure.

According to the study mentioned above, in about 80 per cent of cases an eruption of guttate psoriasis occurs about two to three weeks after a streptococcal infection – commonly referred to as a strep infection. The strep infection usually responsible is tonsillo-pharyngitis, which is commonly referred to as a 'strep' throat. In some cases, you can have 'strep' throat without physical symptoms and it still provokes a bout of guttate psoriasis. When the 'strep' infection has cleared, guttate psoriasis may also clear and not come back. In other people, it does come back, sometimes repeatedly – the likelihood of this increasing if the person is a carrier of the streptococcus bacterium. Sometimes the infection lingers, however, maybe lasting a few weeks or perhaps several months. Unfortunately, a prolonged flare-up of guttate psoriasis can advance into chronic plaque psoriasis – the main form of the disease, as discussed below.

The sudden appearance of guttate psoriasis may be the first experience of psoriasis for some people. On the other hand, it may unexpectedly show itself in a person who has had plaque psoriasis for several years.

Progression to plaque psoriasis

In the study mentioned above, it was found that 68 per cent of patients with guttate psoriasis subsequently developed chronic (long-lasting) plaque psoriasis. The chances of developing chronic plaque psoriasis can be greatly reduced, however, by diligent self-care and by the treatments recommended by your doctor, most of which are described later in this section.

Making the diagnosis

If you suspect that you have guttate psoriasis, you should see your doctor. A diagnosis will be based on the following factors:

- the physical appearance of the rash;
- whether or not the rash was preceded by an infection of some kind;
- whether you have 'ordinary' plaque psoriasis.

If there is still any doubt over the diagnosis, a skin biopsy may be required, where a tiny slice of skin is looked at under a microscope. Before the procedure, you should inform the doctor if you are taking any medications or are allergic to any medications. You may be asked to sign a consent form, too. Apart from that, no special preparations are required.

Blood tests may also be taken to determine whether you have recently had a streptococcal infection.

Treatment

Self-help

As guttate psoriasis usually disappears within a few weeks without medical treatment, regular application of skin softening moisturizers is all that is required. Keeping the skin moist in this way effectively prevents additional irritation. After taking a bath, use thick moisturizers to keep in the moisture and soften the skin.

When the itching is quite troublesome, over-the-counter topical corticosteroids can be used. This is not ideal, however, since there are often numerous individual 'drops' on to which to gently apply the cream.

It is also important to minimize trauma to the skin, caused by scratching, rubbing, bumping or knocking the skin, for example – such trauma can lead to new lesions (or drops) on areas that were previously unaffected.

As guttate psoriasis is so closely linked with streptococcal infection, you can avoid an acute flare-up of symptoms by being watchful for signs of the infection and starting antibiotic treatment early. Most doctors like to prescribe antibiotics to a person with guttate psoriasis as soon as he or she starts to get a sore throat.

Antibiotics

When an outbreak of guttate psoriasis is believed to be linked to a streptococcal infection, you may be prescribed a course of erythromycin, penicillin VK, rifampin or another type of antibiotic. Note that if you have liver problems or are allergic to any of these medicines, you should immediately inform your doctor. Also, be aware that allergic reactions to antibiotics can be serious, even life-threatening – particularly reactions to penicillin.

Phototherapy

Because ultraviolet light can help to clear guttate psoriasis, you may be prescribed a short course of phototherapy, as described in Chapter 7.

PUVA phototherapy is used to treat more resistant cases of guttate psoriasis, and it can effectively clear up the lesions, or bumps. PUVA is a combination of a psoralen drug – this type of drug makes the skin sensitive to sunlight – with exposure to ultraviolet A light, and the drug is taken a few hours before light therapy. Because exposure to the sun after treatment should be avoided, precautions need to be taken to prevent this (by wearing special sunglasses and avoiding going out in the sun). See Chapter 7 for more information on PUVA phototherapy.

In guttate psoriasis, an increase in a certain type of white blood cell (a type of immune cell) called a mast cell has been observed, an increase that is not seen in other forms of psoriasis. The sensitivity of these mast cells to ultraviolet light is believed to be part of the reason that such light clears up lesions.

Narrowband UVB phototherapy is a new treatment which can give similar beneficial results without the need for taking oral medicines.

Surgery

As guttate psoriasis is often linked with streptococcal infection, some doctors will recommend that a person with chronic guttate psoriasis undergo a tonsillectomy – a procedure to remove the tonsils. However, the benefit of tonsillectomy in treating chronic guttate psoriasis was unproven in a series of controlled clinical trials.

Inverse psoriasis

Inverse psoriasis – also called flexural psoriasis – first shows itself as inflamed patches of skin that are smooth and lacking the scales that are associated with plaque psoriasis. These lesions are very red and shiny and are found in folds of the skin that tend to be moist, such as:

- in the armpits
- under the breasts of a woman or heavily built man
- in the genital area (i.e. between the thighs and groin)
- under the buttocks and between each buttock
- beneath the folds of the stomach in an overweight person
- in any other skin folds.

Not every person with inverse psoriasis has lesions in all the above places. The lesions often confine themselves to specific areas, such as under the arms and around the buttocks.

Inverse psoriasis is characterized by a heightened sensitivity to irritation, such as that caused by friction and sweating. It is therefore more frequent and severe in people who are overweight, with deep skin folds (known as flexures). This type of psoriasis can cause a great deal of discomfort, and sexual relations may be difficult for both physical and psychological reasons. In other words, being intimate with a loved one can be not only painful when lesions are present around the genital area, but can cause embarrassment, too.

Treatment

The sensitivity of the skin in the areas affected by this type of psoriasis can make treatment difficult. Some useful treatment regimens include:

- Corticosteroid creams and ointments (see Chapter 5) – in treating inverse psoriasis, topical agents should not be covered with plastic dressings such as cling film (unlike in most other forms of psoriasis). Excessive use of corticosteroid creams, particularly in skin folds, can result in thinning of the skin and stretch marks. Fungal infection may also arise.
- Other topical creams, gels, ointments and so on, such as anthralin or coal tar – although such topical agents can be very effective in treating inverse psoriasis, they can also cause irritation in some people. They should therefore be used with great care under the watchful guidance of a doctor. Moreover, although there is no statistical proof, it is thought that coal tar products may be carcinogenic (cancer-causing).
- Systemic medications (medications that treat the body as a whole) may need to be used for severe inverse psoriasis. See Chapter 6 for more information about systemic medications.
- Some eczema medications such as tacrolimus and pimecrolimus are now being used to treat inverse psoriasis. Dermatologists have discovered that they are often very effective.
- A prescription medication known as Castellani's paint may also be used to treat inverse psoriasis. It is a liquid that can be painted

on to the affected lesions to help dry them up. This product also comes in powder form. Doctors recommend using the powder in the morning and the paint at night.

Erythrodermic psoriasis

This most severe form of psoriasis is caused by the production of more inflammation than is normal in psoriasis. It is by far the least common variant, but affects 85 per cent or more of the body surface and sometimes causes systemic illness – as stated above, 'systemic' means something that involves all of the body's systems (diabetes and hypertension are systemic disorders).

Erythrodermic psoriasis is characterized by a severe reddening of the skin over large areas. The word *erythema* means 'reddening', and *dermic* means 'of the skin'. The condition typically arises in cases of unstable plaque psoriasis where the lesions are not clearly defined. Large, fiery-red patches cover wide areas of skin and, as the skin becomes more livid and begins to shed, there is often severe itching, swelling and pain.

Possible triggers

About 20 per cent of erythrodermic psoriasis cases evolve from plaque psoriasis. It can also be triggered by the following factors:

- infections
- pregnancy
- low calcium levels in the body
- withdrawal of certain oral corticosteroid medications such as prednisone
- stopping the use of strong topical corticosteroids, particularly when they have been used too liberally
- withdrawal of certain other medications, including lithium, interleukin-2 and antimalarial medicines
- strong coal tar preparations.

Similar conditions

Distinguishing certain other skin conditions from generalized erythrodermic psoriasis can be difficult. Similar conditions include:

- allergic reactions to certain drugs
- atopic eczema
- symptoms of lymphoma: a cancer of the lymph nodes.

Treatment

If you begin displaying symptoms of erythrodermic psoriasis, you should seek medical attention straight away.

The initial treatment for erythrodermic psoriasis includes the following:

- topical moisturizers
- the application of cool wet dressings;
- regular oatmeal baths – see page 89
- nutritional support (see Chapter 9)
- bed rest
- low-dose methotrexate, ciclosporin or acitretin (see Chapter 6).

If there is danger of infection, or if an infection is already under way, antibiotics will also be used.

As there is a chance that oral corticosteroids may worsen erythrodermic psoriasis, they should be avoided if possible.

Severe cases

When erythrodermic psoriasis is severe and widespread, the body's ability to control its temperature is disrupted, leading to episodes of shivering and even hypothermia. Protein and fluid loss can also occur, which may result in dehydration and oedema (swelling). Infection may also arise, which can lead to life-threatening illnesses such as pneumonia and even heart failure. Those with this form of psoriasis may require hospital treatment, during which time fluids are put back into the body, the body temperature is stabilized, chemical balances are restored to normal and any infection is treated.

4

The cause of psoriasis

Throughout the long history of psoriasis, scientists have been unable to pinpoint the reason why the skin replaces itself too quickly – the process that underlies all forms of psoriasis. However, in the autumn of 2004, a research team led by Professor Richard Trembath at Leicester University in England made a significant step in the investigation of psoriasis at the important molecular level. For several years, this research team had been involved in a meticulous 'gene hunt', and finally they succeeded in demonstrating that the presence of certain genetic differences in psoriasis means that a person is programmed to be susceptible to developing the condition.

This discovery has been important for the following reasons:

- New and more effectively targeted drugs are now being developed, which is a big step forward.
- The NHS no longer needs to waste money on treatments that are not going to target the right areas.
- It gives doctors a better idea of who may respond to treatment and who may not.
- The person with psoriasis can now appreciate that the disease is not a result of something that he or she has done wrong.

'Susceptibility' genes

Past studies have indicated that 'psoriasis susceptibility genes' are present in a small area of what is known as chromosome 6. Upon closer examination, a gene called CDSN was identified – this gene is responsible for the adhesion (in medicine, 'adhesion' means the abnormal union of surfaces as a result of inflammation or injury) and shedding of skin cells.

Professor Trembath's research team managed to identify the DNA variant of the CDSN gene – and it is this variant that occurs far more frequently in people with psoriasis than it does in unaffected people. Indeed, it makes people more susceptible to developing psoriasis by causing a build-up of CDSN protein. This protein accumulation is believed to contribute to the inflammatory response seen in psoriasis. (See below for more information on inflammation and psoriasis.)

An immune system dysfunction

Scientists have known for a long time that in psoriasis there is an error in the way the immune system works – it is only now that they know the reason. The build-up of protein from the CDSN gene contributes to the abnormal amount of inflammation that is present in psoriasis – indeed, the condition is often referred to an 'inflammatory disease'.

When the immune system is functioning normally, it mobilizes white blood cells when an injury or infection occurs. Masses of white blood cells congregate at the site of the problem, their aim being to rid the body of any foreign invaders such as bacteria or viruses that are taking hold in the area. Immediately, they begin to produce 'factors' capable of repairing wounds, clot the blood and fight any infective agents. It's unfortunate, however, that this process causes the surrounding area to become inflamed and healthy tissue to be injured.

There are two types of white blood cells that come into play to fight foreign substances. They are called lymphocytes and leukocytes. Lymphocytes comprise cells called T cells and B cells, both of which are able to recognize foreign invaders and so launch attacking or defensive action, whichever is appropriate at the time. Helper T cells, known as TH cells, aid them in either fighting or defending, and it is these that scientists have found in high numbers in psoriasis.

An autoimmune problem

Scientists have long had a special interest in TH cells because, when activated, these cells invade the skin cells. Where psoriatic arthritis is concerned, they also infiltrate the joints. The normal action of these TH cells is to stimulate B cells (see above) to produce antibodies – antibodies are proteins that are used by the TH cells to identify and attack foreign substances such as bacteria and viruses. However, in psoriasis, it is auto-antibodies that the TH cells direct the B cells to produce. Auto-antibodies are also known as 'self-antibodies' because the TH cells direct the B cells to fight the body's own cells. In psoriasis, it is skin cells that are attacked by the body's own cells. They start to multiply very rapidly, stacking up on the surface of the skin. (In psoriatic arthritis, it is the cells in the joints that come under attack.) Thereafter, the autoimmune process causes autoimmune antibodies (auto-antibodies) to circulate in the body and maintain the attack, causing the skin cells to continue multiplying rapidly. This is a flare-up of psoriasis and can be present in the same form for a long period or can gradually get worse.

Family history

The presence of a genetic component in psoriasis means that the condition runs in the family – or rather, the *predisposition* to developing psoriasis runs in the family. Indeed, approximately one-third of people with psoriasis have at least one family member with the disease.

Fifty per cent of the genes we carry are inherited from one parent, and 50 per cent are inherited from another, which means that the child of a person with psoriasis has a 25 per cent chance of inheriting the susceptibility, which is a far greater chance than normal. When both parents have psoriasis, the child has a 50 per cent chance of inheriting susceptibility. In twins, if one develops the condition, there is a 70 per cent likelihood that the other will develop it, too. However, because it often doesn't show itself until later in life, statistics aren't always easy to gauge.

So why do some people with a family history of psoriasis never develop it? The clear answer is that a trigger is required, as discussed below. Of the people who apparently have no family members with psoriasis, it is thought that the disease has lain dormant for three or more generations, before which it isn't always easy to have access to the right information. The reason it lies dormant for long periods is believed to be because no trigger is encountered. My brother has psoriatic arthritis and we thought it had come out of the blue. We know now, though, that one of our forebears, maybe in the not-too-distant past, must have had psoriasis in one form or another.

Research has shown that there are two types of plaque psoriasis, one of which tends to develop in young adults and the other of which can develop when a person reaches his or her 50s or 60s. Further research into inherited factors is ongoing.

Trigger factors

A person who is predisposed to getting psoriasis must experience a trigger before the disease process bursts into action. The possible triggers are discussed below. (These things will also trigger a flare-up of psoriasis during a remission.)

Stress and strong emotions

Stress of any kind as well as withheld anger and frustration can have a great impact on the immune system. That is why they are common triggers of psoriasis and its flare-ups. Emotional disorders such as depression and chronic anxiety are strongly linked with flare-ups, too. A study into the effects of stress on a person with psoriasis indicated that, in such a person, stress provokes immune system factors into causing flare-ups.[2]

Infection

The following bacterial and viral infections can trigger psoriasis:

- upper respiratory tract infections caused by the streptococcal bacterium (e.g. tonsillitis, sinusitis and 'strep' throat), which are common triggers of guttate psoriasis (see page 35); ordinary plaque psoriasis can be worsened by such infections, too
- one form of the human papillomavirus (HPV)
- HIV
- *Helicobacter pylori* infection, a common cause of peptic ulcer.

Obesity

The risk of developing inverse psoriasis is increased in people who are overweight. Furthermore, plaques are more likely to develop in the skin folds and creases that are more evident in overweight people.

Injuries to the skin

The skin being knocked, burned or grazed can act as a trigger of plaque psoriasis. Excessive scratching can provoke a flare-up, as can a skin infection or injury by sunburn.

Cold, dry weather

Symptoms often become worse in cold, dry weather and are likely to improve in hot weather and humidity. In addition, sunlight is beneficial for many people; however, it aggravates symptoms in a small minority.

Smoking

Studies have shown that people who smoke tobacco are more susceptible to developing plaque psoriasis. Smoking may also increase the frequency of flare-ups and generally make the disease more severe than it might otherwise have been.

Alcohol

Binge drinking can trigger an attack of psoriasis, as can a regular sustained intake of alcohol.

Certain medications

Symptoms can be worsened by the use of certain drugs, including:

- NSAIDs, such as ibuprofen and naproxen, which are used to reduce inflammation;
- beta-blockers and other drugs used to treat high blood pressure and heart disease;
- progesterone, a female hormone, which is used in the contraceptive pill and other hormonal preparations for women;
- lithium, which is used to treat depression and bipolar disorder;
- antimalarial drugs, such as chloroquine, used to protect against and treat malaria;
- any drug, cream or other preparation that causes a rash as a side effect;
- withdrawal from oral corticosteroids or high-potency corticosteroid creams that cover wide areas of skin – this is known as the 'rebound effect'; there is much concern about this since oral

corticosteroids and corticosteroids creams are, in some cases, used to treat psoriasis.

Whenever you are being prescribed a medication, it's advisable to remind your doctor that you have psoriasis.

Hormonal changes

Changes in hormone levels, particularly in a woman, can cause fluctuations in the severity of psoriasis. For example, the condition is often more severe when hormone levels are high during puberty and when they drop during the menopause. During pregnancy, the severity of symptoms often subsides, and yet in the post-partum period (the six weeks after the baby is born), there is more likely to be an exacerbation of symptoms.

At-risk groups

Psoriasis is often severe in people with weakened immune systems, such as:

- people with autoimmune disorders such as lupus and rheumatoid arthritis;
- people who are HIV-positive – HIV is the virus that causes AIDS; it should be said that as the HIV infection advances, psoriasis generally becomes less active;
- people who are undergoing chemotherapy treatment for cancer.

5

Creams and lotions

Prior to recommending any form of treatment, doctors sometimes work with the patient to set a realistic goal of therapy. As prolonged clearance is seldom achievable – in a 2000 study, this medical belief was proven[3] – it is far better to aim for a reduction of symptoms to a manageable level.

Many people with psoriasis can safely use over-the-counter creams, lotions, ointments and pills, even during flare-ups. It is estimated that only a third of patients with psoriasis require more aggressive prescription therapy. Certain lifestyle changes can help in all cases of psoriasis, but for most they need to be life-long.

Unfortunately, there is always the capacity for a medication – whether bought over the counter or acquired by prescription – to cause side effects. You should therefore monitor your reaction very carefully. It is important to note that a treatment for psoriasis should never be worse than the psoriasis itself.

In general there are three treatment options for psoriasis, as described below:

1 *Topical medications* – i.e. those that are applied only to the surface of the skin. These include lotions, creams and shampoos and are generally the first line of fire for mild to moderate psoriasis. They rarely completely clear the problem, but they can often reduce symptoms to a level you can cope with.
2 *Phototherapy.* The options here include light-wave radiation using broad or narrow band ultraviolet B (UVB) or the drug psoralen with ultraviolet A (known as PUVA). It is known that moderate to severe psoriasis responds fairly well to this treatment, which is obviously good news. Phototherapy treatments are more effective than drugs and carry fewer side effects than the majority of systemic agents. Phototherapy is discussed in greater detail in Chapter 7.

3 *Systemic agents* – i.e. those that treat the whole body and not just the skin. There are various treatments under this category, and they are usually reserved for severe psoriasis since they can cause significant side effects. Systemic agents are often combined with phototherapy and are discussed in greater detail in Chapter 6.

In order to establish which treatments are the safest and most effective, controlled comparison studies need to be carried out. Every case is different and doctors must discuss treatment options with the patient, taking into effect his or her individual requirements. If you feel that your doctor is giving you insufficient information or prescribing treatments without first taking your needs and opinions into account, it is important that you speak up and let your wishes be known.

As with all medications, your doctor needs to know if you are pregnant or breastfeeding or if you are planning to become pregnant during the course of your psoriasis treatment.

Over-the-counter topical treatments

The dry skin that comes with mild to moderate psoriasis – particularly plaque psoriasis – will often benefit from the use of topical treatments that are mostly available without a doctor's prescription. Keeping the skin moist and lubricated is an essential basic treatment approach. Creams and ointments are more effective for some people than others. If one preparation fails to be of help, ask your doctor to recommend a different one.

Emollients

Emollients are preparations that soften the skin. They are available as:

- *E45 cream* – this emollient contains a blend of mineral oils and zinc oxide, which help to soften skin. Because soap can be very drying, E45 cream should be used in its place for washing and bathing. Avoid contact with the eyes.
- *Cetraben cream* – this emollient is made from liquid paraffin and glycerine. It works by placing a layer of oil on the skin's surface

to prevent fluids from evaporating. The best results are achieved when used daily in combination with a good-quality moisturizing cream, such as aqueous cream.

Moisturizers

Moisturizers effectively reduce fluid loss from the outer layer of the skin and so help to hydrate it, limiting dryness and scaling. After 'washing' with an emollient, a good moisturizing cream should be applied. Aqueous cream is highly recommended in this respect as it is cheap and non-greasy and it can be purchased in bulk. It should be applied liberally and frequently, depending on how dry the skin is. Aqueous cream is used to great effect by many people with psoriasis.

Coal tar

Coal tar is obtained by distilling coal at very high temperatures. It is a brown or black liquid that is thick and gluey, with a distinctive smell. When combined with other ingredients such as salicylic or lactic acid, it can be manufactured into creams, lotions, gels, shampoos and ointments. Coal tar is available over the counter and, at higher potency, as a prescription medication. How coal tar works is not completely understood, but it appears to have antiseptic and anti-itching properties that are capable of normalizing keratin growth in the skin and so reducing the scaling effect of psoriasis. Coal tar has been a treatment of psoriasis, eczema (including atopic dermatitis) and other skin conditions for many years, often proving very successful. Coal tar preparations contain many thousands of different compounds, as a result of which no two batches are composed of exactly the same ingredients, and some batches are more effective than others.

There is some concern over whether coal tar products have carcinogenic (cancer-causing) properties – some studies found a raised risk of skin cancer in animals. However, there has not been one human link in 75 years of documented use. If you are worried about the risk, you may prefer not to use coal tar products, or to use them only as a last resort if other products fail.

How to use coal tar therapies

A coal tar preparation should be left on the skin for at least two hours. It is best to apply it at bedtime and leave it on overnight – in that way you reduce the inconvenience of coping with the smell. If you are using it as a shampoo to treat scalp psoriasis, work it in with downward strokes, in the same direction as the hair grows. Finally, cover or wrap with bandages to help the preparation to stay in place and minimize staining. Avoid covering with plastic wrap (cling film) as, in this case, it encourages irritation and infection. If the area is infected, raw, blistered or oozing, don't apply this treatment.

Coal tar treatments are usually tolerated very well. There may be the following side effects, however:

- initial mild stinging which usually settles down as your body grows accustomed to the treatment – if the stinging continues, stop the treatment and ask your doctor's advice;
- temporary discoloration on bleached, tinted, blond or grey hair;
- staining of the skin – it will return to normal once the treatment has been stopped;
- staining of clothes, towels and so on;
- photosensitivity – in other words, the eyes may hurt in bright sunlight and the chances of getting sunburnt may be greater.

Ingesting coal tar is dangerous, even life-threatening, and emergency treatment should be sought without delay if a coal tar preparation has been swallowed.

Topical corticosteroids

Topical (meaning 'applied to the skin') corticosteroids, such as halobetasol, are the mainstay of psoriasis treatments; they range in strength from very mild to very strong and come in the form of solutions, gels, creams, lotions, sprays, ointments and foam. These preparations have powerful anti-inflammatory properties that suppress the immune system and slow the turnover of skin cells, thereby reducing inflammation and itching.

The risks of using corticosteroids

The problem with corticosteroids is that although they are great at reducing inflammation, they don't seem to have any real healing effect on the skin. Moreover, when you stop applying them, the problem can quickly reappear, and sometimes with more ferocity than ever. However, although this is a risk, it doesn't happen enough to stop doctors from prescribing them. In short, the benefits generally outweigh the risks.

Another concern is that anything rubbed into the skin is absorbed into the bloodstream. The corticosteroids in these preparations are synthetic replications of the corticosteroid hormones that we produce naturally in our bodies and as such they may fool the body into reducing its own output of corticosteroids. There is one vital hormone called hydrocortisone, which we require in order to cope with stress. For as long as someone is using the cream there is often no change, but as soon as its use is stopped the body's reserves of hydrocortisone may drop. This could pose a real danger, particularly if the person concerned is faced with an emergency of some kind. However, this is a very slight risk and is only a concern where high-potency corticosteroid cream is applied to very large areas of the body for a long period of time.

With the risks in mind, low-strength corticosteroid creams and ointments are often recommended for sensitive areas and for widespread patches of damaged skin. Stronger corticosteroid preparations may be prescribed for smaller areas of skin and any stubborn plaques on your hands and feet. Also, they are often used on active outbreaks until they are under control.

Strong corticosteroids should not be used continuously for long periods of time. Indeed, a two-week cycle of treatment with twice-daily applications is normally recommended. However, recent studies have suggested that once-daily treatment may be more effective. Ask your doctor about this, and follow the instruction leaflet very carefully. During a flare-up of mild to moderate psoriasis, fast relief may be obtained by the use of a high-potency topical corticosteroid, often in combination with an oral medication.

Certain corticosteroids such as triamcinolone can be delivered by injection to treat nail psoriasis.

When using topical corticosteroids, carefully follow your doctor's advice.

Side effects on the skin

After a period of using corticosteroids, there is a chance of the following effects on the skin:

- Fine, downy hair may grow.
- Acne spots may develop, particularly when the cream is used under an airtight adhesive bandage.
- The skin may become very thin, showing obvious stretch marks or turning bright red.
- If very thin, the skin may be easily damaged, so that an apparently minor injury can cause a nasty gash. Knocks and bumps can lead to heavy bruising.
- There is a small chance of infection occurring.

Although these effects may appear worrying, none of them is serious. On cessation of treatment, the skin usually returns to how it was, with the exception of stretch marks in some people.

Pregnancy and breastfeeding

As high-potency corticosteroids have been shown to carry a small risk of adrenal insufficiency, this type of medication should not be used in pregnancy and breastfeeding. Adrenal insufficiency means that the body loses its ability to produce natural corticosteroid hormones for a length of time after the drug has been withdrawn, with serious complications. This event is uncommon and, with topical corticosteroids, usually mild – but your doctor will probably want you to err on the side of caution and steer clear of them if you are pregnant or breastfeeding or if you are intending to get pregnant.

Rebound flare-up

A 'rebound' flare-up of psoriasis can occur when corticosteroid treatments are stopped abruptly. It is therefore best to reduce their use slowly. Only use topical corticosteroids on your face and other sensitive areas if instructed to do so by your doctor. Avoid getting them in your eyes.

Corticosteroids for scalp psoriasis

There are several prescription-only topical corticosteroid medications that are specifically aimed at treating scalp psoriasis, as discussed in detail in Chapter 3. They contain clobetasol propionate, which is often very effective at clearing psoriasis.

It is possible for some cases of scalp psoriasis to become resistant to topical corticosteroids. Fortunately there are other available treatments, such as anthralin and tar.

Anthralin

Anthralin, when applied to psoriasis plaques, can slow down the division of skin cells. It inhibits DNA replication, preventing the skin cells from multiplying excessively. As a result, the thickening and scaling of skin is reduced, inflammation is decreased and the skin becomes smooth. It can produce a remission that lasts for months. However, because it can also stain the skin and cause local burning and irritation, short contact anthralin therapy (SCAT) is mainly used, in which it is applied to the skin for a short time every day. Leave it on for no more than 20 minutes, then wash it off with lukewarm water. It's important to note that a first application should stay on for no more than 10 minutes. There is 1% cream with which to begin your treatment and a 3% cream for thereafter. If irritation occurs after using the 3% cream, you should go back to using the 1% cream. Your hands should be washed thoroughly after use.

Anthralin is used mainly to treat chronic or inactive psoriasis rather than acute or inflamed outbreaks. However, over the past few years its use has declined with the launch of the vitamin D topical compounds, one example of which is calcipotriene, as discussed below.

Anthralin is available as a cream, ointment, paste and soap. The soap can be used to wash your hair, but great care must be taken not to get it into your eyes. If your skin becomes stained, it will fade in two or three weeks. Take care not to stain clothes, towels, bed linen and so on because it may not wash out. It is best to wear old clothes, use old towels and even put on old bed linen that you don't mind being stained.

This medication should not be used in the following instances:

- for treating young children and infants
- in pustular psoriasis
- on broken, inflamed, oozing or blistered skin
- near the face, in skin folds or around the genitals.

Inform your doctor if you are pregnant or breastfeeding.

Vitamin D compounds

The Dead Sea in Israel has become a modern mecca for psoriasis treatment, and thousands of psoriasis patients every year sunbathe nude at its shores. Why the Dead Sea? It's because special receptors in the skin allow vitamin D, which is generated by sunlight exposure, to penetrate and become activated by a hormone that stops cells from growing and shedding too quickly. Sunlight exposure is therefore of great benefit to most people with psoriasis, and the low elevation of the Dead Sea stops the harshest of sun rays from damaging the skin, allowing sunbathers to stay out for longer without burning.

Vitamin D, when applied to the skin as an ointment or shampoo, not only slows down skin cell growth, it also reduces itching and inflammation. It is therefore a useful topical treatment, of benefit for scalp psoriasis as well as other forms of the condition.

Calcipotriene

Calcipotriene – also known as calcipotriol – contains a synthetic form of vitamin D (known as vitamin D3) and is available as a cream, ointment or solution for treating mild to moderate psoriasis. It is proving very popular because it doesn't stain and is at least as effective as anthralin and coal tar treatments. Therefore, it is more commonly prescribed. There is now also a foam preparation which makes it even easier to use.

Calcipotriene does not give as much benefit as the highest potency corticosteroids, but products and regimens that combine both compounds are more effective than either compound in isolation. The following are good examples:

- a cream that contains both calcipotriene and betamethasone, which can be of more benefit than either compound alone;
- vitamin D ointments in combination with phototherapy treatment, which can be useful;
- vitamin D ointments combined with oral therapies such as methotrexate, acitretin or ciclosporin, which can increase effectiveness and allow lower doses of either medication, reducing the possibility of side effects.

There are possible side effects:

- Skin irritation occurs in about 20 per cent of cases, a higher rate than for people using potent corticosteroids. You may be able to dilute the agent with petroleum to prevent this problem – speak to your doctor about this. It is also advisable to avoid using the agent on or near to sensitive areas such as the face and folds of skin.
- In children, there is concern that it may lower levels of vitamin D to the extent that it has a negative impact on bone growth.
- When applied to large areas of skin, a condition known as hypercalcaemia (very high levels of calcium in the blood) may occur.

Topical retinoids

Topical retinoids are vitamin A derivatives that appear to normalize the activity of DNA in the skin cells. They were originally developed to treat acne and severe sunburn; however, tazarotene is a retinoid that was formulated specifically to treat psoriasis and is available in gel or cream form.

Unlike oral retinoids, tazarotene is of benefit to the affected skin tissue without causing systemic problems (i.e. problems affecting the whole of the body), such as aching and tiredness. There is also no thinning of the skin or tolerance to the drug, as occurs with corticosteroids. A very small amount is required on each area, which can include the scalp and nails if needed. When using the gel, no more than 20 per cent of the body should be covered at one time, and when using the cream, no more than 35 per cent should be covered – the palm of the hand represents about one per cent of the body surface.

To avoid any resulting dryness and irritation, you can apply either zinc oxide or a moisturizer around the treated area. If severe skin irritation occurs, your doctor will probably recommend that you use it in combination with another treatment, which allows a lower dose. You may be able to mix it in equal amounts with petroleum jelly, gradually increasing the amount of tazarotene to encourage the skin to become less sensitive – but ask your doctor about this.

When combined with another therapy such as topical corticosteroids or phototherapy, topical retinoids are more effective.

Pregnancy and breastfeeding

As vitamin A derivatives have been linked with birth defects, topical retinoids should be avoided in pregnancy and breastfeeding. If you are pregnant or breastfeeding or if you are wishing to become pregnant, it is essential that you inform your doctor.

Salicylic acid

Salicylic acid is the active agent in aspirin. As a topical cream, it can help to remove scaly plaque. Note that if it is used on large areas of the body, nausea and ringing in the ears can occur – therefore it should be applied to small areas only. Owing to its great ability to enhance other agents, it can be combined with high-potency corticosteroids such as clobetasol propionate, betamethasone and furoate. Your doctor will tell you about this.

Combination therapy

Topical medications are often most effective when used in combination with another treatment. For instance, the following commonly used combination therapy works very well as a maintenance regime: a high-potency, oral corticosteroid medication such as halobetasol (see page 52), taken only at the weekend, plus the topical agent calcipotriene, used twice daily on weekdays only.

Your doctor will know whether to recommend that you use combination therapy, and will advise you about what to do.

How to use a cream

When using a cream or ointment, it is important to follow the instructions that come with it very carefully. The pointers below should also help:

- As it is the layer of cream that is actually touching the skin that does the most good, it is not necessary to slap on a thick coating.
- It is also less wasteful to limit the cream to the affected area only, avoiding contact with healthy skin.
- Scoop a blob of cream on to your finger, place it on the affected area and gently rub in, being careful to cover the entire area.

When a topical agent can be combined with phototherapy (see Chapter 7 for more information on phototherapy), it is even more important that you follow the instructions. Light rays will obviously have more difficulty penetrating a thick layer than a thin layer of cream before reaching your skin. If you apply a thick layer you will not reap the maximum reward.

When using a topical treatment, the following precautions should be upheld:

- Don't use any old cream given you by your friends and relatives. Their intentions may be good, but many creams contain powerful toxic ingredients that would do more harm than good. If you are keen to try a particular cream, be sure to ask your doctor's advice first of all.
- Keep a record of all the creams and ointments that you have used, noting the name of each one, how long you used it, how much benefit it gave you and the dates you used it. This may come in useful if your doctor is considering recommending a new topical treatment.

Occlusive dressings

Tapes or wrappings that are occlusive – meaning that they are airtight and watertight – can help psoriasis wounds, such as gashes and cuts, to heal. As well as protecting against abrasion and irritation, they keep water out and allow sweat to stay in, which helps to return moisture to the area and prevent scaling. Occlusive dressings are particularly useful for wounds on the palms of the hands and soles of the feet.

In some cases, it can be very helpful to apply a corticosteroid cream beneath a high-potency corticosteroid tape. Alternatively, it is possible to use a tape (such as Cordran tape) that is already impregnated with a potent corticosteroid such as flurandrenolide, which can prove highly beneficial. In studies, tapes impregnated with a high-potency corticosteroid are proving more successful than high-potency corticosteroid creams alone.

There are possible drawbacks of using a tape impregnated with a high-potency corticosteroid:

- The tape can be expensive.
- There is a greater chance of skin irritation than when using the cream alone.
- After cessation of use, there is a greater risk of rebound effects than when using the cream alone.
- Corticosteroid-impregnated tapes heighten the risk of secondary infections. This can be avoided by changing the tapes every 12 hours.
- When using the tape on large areas, there is a risk of a disorder known as adrenal insufficiency. This can be serious as it causes the body to lose its ability to produce natural steroids.

You should never use a corticosteroid cream beneath occlusive tape without your doctor's agreement.

6

Pills and injections

Treatments given by mouth (orally) and administered by injection enter the whole body and its systems (not just the skin) and are therefore referred to by doctors as 'systemic'. When a substance gains access into an entire system, it exerts an effect – sometimes profound, sometimes minuscule – on every part of it. In the case of a medicine, some of the effects are positive whereas some are negative. Obviously, the positive must be seen to outdo the negative or there is no point in using it.

Topical treatments are usually the first line of defence in treating psoriasis (as discussed in Chapter 5), whereas agents taken by mouth or administered by injection are far more powerful and are reserved for severe and incapacitating cases of psoriasis – ones that fail to respond to the less potent creams, lotions and other topical therapies. Their benefits are often greater than when topical agents are used in isolation, but they come with some potentially serious side effects. Systemic agents are often used in conjunction with topical treatments to achieve a better outcome.

The systemic treatments methotrexate, the oral retinoids and ciclosporin are licensed to treat psoriasis and usually offer the best results. They also carry a lower risk of side effects and so can be described as first-line therapies. Second-line therapy involves drugs that are commonly used for psoriasis but that are not specifically licensed to treat the condition even though they have been found to be effective – such drugs include hydroxyurea (also known as hydroxycarbamide), sulfasalazine, tioguanine, mofetil, azathioprine and oral tacrolimus. Unfortunately, these agents are more potent and therefore carry a greater risk of side effects.

Obviously, the first-line therapies are used first of all in psoriasis treatment, but, if the treatment is unsatisfactory for some reason, it is possible to fall back on the second-line therapies. Within the confines of this book it is not possible for me to go into detail about the many second-line therapies available, since many drugs that are licensed for the treatment of other conditions have been found to be of benefit in psoriasis.

First-line therapies include:

- methotrexate (an immunosuppressant drug)
- oral retinoids (synthetic forms of vitamin A)
- ciclosporin (an immunosuppressant drug).

The second-line therapies that are most commonly used (although carrying the risk of more side effects than the first-line therapies) include:

- sulfasalazine
- hydroxyurea (also known as hydroxycarbamide)
- tioguanine.

Methotrexate

Some experts believe that severe widespread plaque psoriasis responds better to a DMARD called methotrexate than to any other therapy. It certainly gives excellent results. In fact, one treatment centre announced that, after taking methotrexate, 80 per cent of its psoriasis patients reported prolonged improvement – a fine response indeed. Methotrexate is also of great benefit for patients with psoriatic arthritis and other severe forms of the disease, including pustular and erythrodermic psoriasis. Moreover, people with acute exacerbations of otherwise stable psoriasis often respond well to short-term use of methotrexate, as indicated in a study in which both methotrexate and ciclosporin were tested.[4] (See page 67 for more information on the drug ciclosporin.)

Methotrexate works by blocking an enzyme called dihydrofolate reductase, and this blockage has the effect of hindering the production of folic acid. Folic acid is involved in the creation of skin cells, blood cells, gastrointestinal tissue cells and immune system cells. As a result, the overgrowth of skin cells is halted and inflammation goes down.

Methotrexate is usually taken orally, in tablet form. However, injections may be administered when higher doses are needed or to reduce side effects. The drug should be taken exactly as directed, improvements normally being seen between three and six weeks after commencing treatment.

Folic acid

As methotrexate effectively inhibits the metabolism of folic acid, some people using methotrexate develop a deficiency in this substance, which can produce the following symptoms:

- nausea or vomiting (or both)
- headache
- rash
- diarrhoea
- mouth sores (stomatitis)
- slight hair loss – hair grows back when the medication is stopped
- muscle aches.

Although most people are not troubled at all by side effects, those who are usually find that they disappear over time. If they happen to persist, you can find relief by taking folate supplements in the form of B complex vitamins. Your doctor may prescribe these.

Where there is a more serious shortfall of folic acid – not able to be sufficiently restored by vitamin B supplementation – there is obviously a greater risk of more serious complications. However, they are more likely to occur at higher doses of the drug. The possible complications of severe folic acid deficiency include:

- severe anaemia – folic acid supplementation can combat this;
- infections, particularly shingles (herpes zoster) and pneumonia;
- kidney complications;
- liver damage such as cirrhosis and scarring – people with existing liver problems should not take methotrexate; in other people, liver function tests (a type of blood test) should be carried out on a regular basis;
- bone marrow toxicity, causing suppression of blood cell production;
- problems in the reproductive process – methotrexate can trigger a miscarriage or cause birth defects, so it should not be taken in

pregnancy or if you are planning to get pregnant. There is also a possibility of impaired fertility in men;

- bone density loss and osteoporosis;
- lung disease, with sudden onset – although this complication is rare, occurring in less than 5 per cent of people who take methotrexate, it is a very serious matter. The people most at risk are the elderly and those who have protein in the urine or diabetes. People with existing rheumatoid problems or who have ever taken DMARDs – drugs that treat rheumatoid arthritis – are also at risk of lung disease so should not take methotrexate. Any lung-related symptoms such as coughing or shortness of breath should be reported to your doctor.

As a deficiency in folic acid does not necessarily produce symptoms, anyone taking methotrexate should have routine blood tests every 8–12 weeks.

Drug interactions

Certain drugs are capable of interacting with methotrexate, which can cause toxicity problems. For instance, the antibiotic trimethoprim–sulfamethoxazole increases the toxicity of methotrexate. NSAIDs such as aspirin, ibuprofen and naproxen can also cause toxicity problems and should be avoided, if possible. It is important to note that people with psoriatic arthritis can safely take the NSAIDs ketoprofen, fluorobiprofen and piroxicam.

Sunlight

The skin can become more sensitive to sunlight when you are taking methotrexate, so use plenty of sunscreen when you go out.

Alcohol

As the risk of liver damage increases when taking methotrexate, it is best to cut out alcohol completely. If it is difficult to do this at special occasions – weddings and other celebrations, for example – try to have just one drink. Medical opinion is that it is safest to have no more than one alcoholic beverage per month when taking methotrexate.

Drug interactions

It is important that you inform your doctor of all the medications that you are taking. When taking methotrexate, certain interactions are possible:

- The toxicity of methotrexate may be increased by the antibiotic trimethoprim, which is used to treat urinary and respiratory infections.
- NSAIDs may affect the level of methotrexate in the blood. You should therefore be closely monitored when taking NSAIDs.
- Over-the-counter drugs and natural remedies may increase the toxicity of methotrexate. It is therefore important that you keep your doctor fully informed of all that you are taking.
- As vaccinations can react adversely with methotrexate, ask your doctor's advice if a vaccine needs to be administered.

Oral retinoids

Oral retinoids, which are derived from vitamin A, are basically suppressive agents that are often used in the treatment of psoriasis. They have the following properties:

- They have an anti-inflammatory effect.
- They help to calm down the overproduction of cells.
- They can benefit the arthritis that may arise with psoriasis.

The oral retinoids of most benefit in treating psoriasis include acitretin and isotretinoin. However, acitretin is by far the most widely used.

As this type of drug only suppresses the condition, long-term treatment is often required.

Acitretin

When acitretin is used in severe psoriasis – particularly the pustular or erythrodermic forms – the clearance can appear dramatic. Acitretin is often of a little less benefit against more common forms such as plaque or guttate psoriasis, particularly when used alone, but every case is different and the responses vary a great deal. For instance, when given alone as a treatment for the more common forms of psoriasis, acitretin was shown in a study to produce 66 per cent clearance after 24 weeks,[5] whereas in a study carried out the following year there was 80 per cent clearance after only 12 weeks.[6] General usage of acitretin has indicated that, as a solo treatment, it can be expected to produce around a 70 per cent clearance in approximately eight weeks.

Because acitretin is easily absorbed and widely distributed around the body, it is often combined with other agents such as topical creams or PUVA phototherapy (see Chapter 7) to produce a more substantial improvement. In general, acitretin combined with PUVA and UVB phototherapy enables faster and more thorough results, requiring lower doses of radiation, which, in turn, reduces the risk of side effects in the skin and mucous membranes.

It is important to note that because acitretin can trigger a miscarriage, foetal death and serious birth defects, women of childbearing age should take it only under a doctor's recommendation. See page 58 for more information about oral retinoids and pregnancy.

Isotretinoin

Although isotretinoin is not nearly so potent as acitretin, it is often used successfully as a treatment of pustular psoriasis. It can also benefit pustular psoriasis when used in conjunction with phototherapy.

As with acitretin, it is vitally important to note that isotretinoin should not be taken during pregnancy or when a pregnancy is planned. There is a risk of miscarriage, early foetal death or serious birth defects.

Side effects of oral retinoids

Oral retinoids are among the safest of the systemic therapies for psoriasis. Even so, there are possible side effects and potentially serious toxicity reactions, including:

- If oral retinoids are taken during pregnancy, there is a significant risk of birth defects.
- There can be problems with the skin and mucous membranes. The latter are the sensitive areas contiguous with the skin, such as the delicate tissues inside the nostrils, sinuses, ears, lips,

genital region and anus. The thick, sticky fluid secreted by some of the mucous membranes is termed mucus. As a result of taking oral retinoids, a dry nose, dry eyes, chapped lips, nosebleeds, dry 'sticky-feeling' skin, peeling palms and soles and thinning hair can occur. These problems are often relieved by taking daily supplements of vitamin E.

- There may be fatigue, joint pain, bruising and headaches.
- Eye problems can occur, including blurred vision, conjunctivitis, cataracts and poorer night vision.
- There is a greater risk of excess bone growth, particularly at the ankles, knees and pelvic area.
- The blood level of triglycerides can be raised. Triglycerides are fatty molecules (lipids) in the blood that can lead to atherosclerosis – a disease of the arteries causing heart attack and stroke. This may be prevented by the use of cholesterol-lowering agents, such as gemfibrozil or statins, an example being atovastatin.
- There is a very slight risk of a condition occurring in the brain called benign intracranial hypertension (pseudotumor cerebri). The symptoms linked to this disorder are headache, blurred vision, nausea and vomiting. If you experience these symptoms, stop taking the retinoid and seek emergency treatment. Isotretinoin appears to be more likely than acitretin to cause this problem.
- Liver damage is also a risk, which is why regular blood tests should be taken to measure enzyme levels.
- Isotretinoin has been linked with depression and, in a small number of patients, suicidal feelings.

To minimize the risk of side effects, experts recommend a low-fat diet with fish oil supplements and plenty of exercise, including aerobic exercise.

Ciclosporin

The drug ciclosporin (sometimes spelt 'cyclosporine') can effectively treat all forms of psoriasis. It is an immunosuppressant, meaning it is capable of decreasing immune system activity. As a result, it is often used after organ transplants to reduce the risk of rejection. Because long-term use of ciclosporin can cause significant toxicity problems, including kidney problems and non-melanoma skin cancers (see below for further possible side effects), it is best used to treat acute (short-term) situations. In psoriasis, short-term use is usually very effective – indeed, taking ciclosporin for as little as five days to treat acute psoriasis can give rapid control, with a lower risk of side effects. A switch to other, long-term, treatments is then often recommended.

Ciclosporin use is reserved for patients who fail to respond to phototherapy or less potent systemic therapies such as metho-trexate or acitretin. The brand of ciclosporin usually used is Neural, which has a success rate in psoriasis of 60–91 per cent. The use of this drug is usually limited to one year, but some experts believe it is safe for up to two years. Seek your doctor's advice about this.

Because ciclosporin is an immune system suppressant, it is not offered to patients with active infections and cancer. Ciclosporin can cause problems for people with uncontrolled high blood pressure or impaired kidney function and therefore patients considered for ciclosporin therapy are given a thorough health check before-hand. For instance, blood pressure and blood levels of creatinine should be within normal bounds. (Creatinine is a breakdown compound excreted in the urine, the levels of which may indicate renal dysfunction.) If blood pressure is raised during ciclosporin therapy, the dose is usually reduced by about 30 per cent and antihyperten-sive medications prescribed. Some experts believe that hypertensive medications can worsen psoriasis, in which case calcium-channel blockers may be used. It is best to ask your doctor's advice about this.

The common and usually temporary side effects associated with ciclosporin include fatigue, joint pain, headaches, tremor, gingivitis and body hair growth. The more serious complications include:

- kidney damage – prolonged use of ciclosporin always causes injury to the kidneys;
- high blood pressure, as discussed above;
- raised cholesterol and lipid levels, which should be treated with cholesterol-lowering agents;
- increased risk of infections;

- raised levels of calcium and low levels of magnesium – these problems can be remedied by taking magnesium supplements and eating a diet rich in potassium;
- liver abnormalities;
- skin cancers – there is a higher than normal incidence of carcinoma in patients who have taken ciclosporin after PUVA phototherapy;
- lymphoma (cancer of the lymph nodes).

Sulfasalazine

Sulfasalazine is a systemic agent with anti-inflammatory properties. It is used to reduce symptoms in a range of inflammatory disorders. It is may also be the medication of choice for psoriasis, used alone or in combination with other treatments. Sulfasalazine and methotrexate are the only drugs that have been proved effective for treating psoriatic arthritis.

Your doctor needs to know whether you drink alcohol, and if so how much, whether you drink caffeine, and whether you smoke tobacco or use illegal drugs – these things may affect the way the medication functions. In addition, tell your doctor if you have ever experienced asthma, anaemia or another blood disorder, intestinal or urinary tract obstruction, kidney disease, liver disease, severe allergies or porphyria (a condition caused by abnormal metabolism of haemoglobin).

Side effects

Unfortunately, owing to its side effects, some people are forced to stop using sulfasalazine. The most common side effects include headaches, diarrhoea, dizziness, indigestion and nausea. If you have any of these side effects and they become bothersome they should be reported to your doctor.

Possible side effects requiring medical attention include:

- chest pain
- fever, chills or sore throat
- difficulty breathing, wheezing
- difficulty swallowing

- unusual bleeding or bruising
- bloody diarrhoea
- skin rash
- joint or muscle aches
- redness, blistering, peeling or loosening of the skin, including inside the mouth
- a cold that fails to improve
- yellowing of the eyes or skin
- pale skin
- unusual weakness or tiredness
- stomach cramps
- painful or reduced urination.

Blood problems

Many of the above-mentioned symptoms arise from blood problems – a constant risk in sulfasalazine therapy. It is therefore essential that you have your blood checked on a regular basis. Remember to inform your doctor if you experience any of the symptoms listed above.

Sunlight and ultraviolet rays

As sulfasalazine can make your skin more sensitive to ultraviolet light or sunlight exposure, try to keep out of the sun or wear protective clothing and a sunscreen with a sun protection factor of at least 15. Avoid using sun lamps or sun tanning beds.

Hydroxyurea (also known as hydroxycarbamide)

Hydroxyurea is licensed as a chemotherapy drug and used to treat some forms of cancer. It has also been found to be of benefit in treating moderate to severe psoriasis because it can effectively slow down the rapid division of skin cells. It is generally not so effective as many other psoriasis therapies but it can be used with phototherapy treatments. The downside to the drug is its often untenable side effects, which may even be life-threatening. For that reason it must be prescribed with good judgement and used with great caution.

If you have ever had a blood disease such as anaemia or leukaemia, or if you have ever had gout, make sure that your doctor is aware of that fact.

The most common side effects include the following:

- Lowered resistance to infection – as hydroxyurea (hydroxy-carbamide) can decrease the production of white blood cells, there is more chance of infection occurring. Seek medical advice if you experience the feverishness and body aches associated with a viral infection, or the localized heat, swelling, redness and pain associated with a bacterial infection.
- Anaemia (reduced haemoglobin) – see your doctor if you feel tired and breathless.
- Raised levels of uric acid in the blood – apart from gout, which can occur with raised levels of uric acid, there are few physical pointers to the presence of abnormal levels of uric acid. For this reason, you will have regular blood tests while taking this drug. Drinking plenty of fluids can help to stop this problem.

The less common side effects (shown below) usually subside between seven and 21 days after starting treatment. If you find them excessive or unbearable, speak to your doctor. There may be another therapy that suits you better, or a treatment that encourages the symptom to calm down. These less common side effects include:

- nausea and vomiting
- sore mouth and mouth ulcers
- food tasting different
- diarrhoea
- hair loss
- skin rash.

Biologic response modifiers

Biologic response modifiers – commonly described as 'biologics' – are different from most drugs in that they are derived from living human or animal proteins (hence the name 'biologic'). In today's world, it is far more common for drugs to be developed by combining specific chemical substances. However, biologics have qualities that chemical drugs do not have.

Biologics have been around for over 100 years, but it is only recently that scientists have been able to target them at the underlying problems in psoriasis and psoriatic arthritis. They are therefore now viewed as the most exciting development in psoriasis treatment.

Most psoriasis treatments, phototherapy included, target the immune system in some way, but because their impact is broad, there is always the risk of damage to other areas of the body. Biologics, however, are more able to target specific psoriasis trouble-spots within the immune system. This makes them a safer option, sparing the body of broad side effects. In short, biologics carry a low risk of side effects, whereas there is a greater risk of side effects from chemical drugs. You may wonder, then, why biologics aren't offered as a matter of course to everyone with psoriasis. The answer is that they are expensive medications to produce and are not at all easy to use. Indeed, they must be administered by injection or intravenous infusion, as discussed below.

How do biologics work?

Biologics work specifically on overactive immune system components – some of which are the T cells and some the chemical messengers released by T cells. It is the job of T cells to recognize viruses, bacteria and other potentially harmful agents and lead the immune system in attacking and destroying them. In psoriasis, some of the T cells mount an attack for no reason, migrating upwards to the skin where they behave as though fighting an infection or healing a wound – the end result being the rapid over-production of skin cells and the creation of plaques. Biologics are able to prevent the activation or migration of T cells.

Administration of biologics

One type of biologic is administered by infusion but most types are given by intramuscular injection or subcutaneous injection. An injection of this type of drug is usually administered by a doctor. However, with training and advice, most types can be self-administered in the comfort of your own home, although intravenous infusions must always be delivered under medical care.

After an injection or infusion, it is possible to experience flu-like symptoms or to develop an infection at the injection site. Such side effects are generally mild, short-lived and not sufficiently troublesome to stop the person from taking the medication. It should be added that, in a few cases, an allergic reaction to the injection can occur, which is why doctors prefer to administer the injection themselves, within an environment that is best equipped for such an eventuality.

Whether any long-term problems can arise from taking biologics is still not known – they are a relatively new group of drugs and their safety continues to be assessed.

Biologics used to treat psoriasis

The following biologics are used for psoriasis:

- *Etanercept* is used to treat moderate to severe plaque psoriasis and to improve physical function in psoriatic arthritis. Etanercept can either be given alone or in conjunction with methotrexate. Patients inject themselves under the skin (subcutaneously), once or twice weekly for 12 weeks. This drug should not be used if you have a weakened immune system or heart disease.
- *Efalizumab* is used to treat moderate to severe plaque psoriasis. Patients can inject themselves at home under the skin (subcutaneously), once weekly for 12 weeks. Clinical trials have indicated that a 24-week course of injection treatment can be equally safe and produce better plaque clearance. After stopping this treatment, some people experience a flare-up of lesions.
- *Infliximab* is used to treat psoriatic arthritis. This medication is delivered once a week by intravenous infusion during the initial six weeks of treatment, after which one infusion is given every eight weeks. The infusions are given in a hospital or medical centre and last for two hours. Infliximab should not be used if you are suffering from heart disease.

The National Institute for Health and Clinical Excellence (NICE) advises that etanercept should be the first biologic offered in severe psoriasis and psoriatic arthritis. If there is no marked improvement after 12 weeks, the treatment should be stopped and one of the other biologics offered.

Who can use biologics?

Biologic medications may be offered to people in the following groups:

- Those with severe and intolerable plaque psoriasis or psoriatic arthritis (or both) who have failed to respond to other systemic treatments (such as PUVA phototherapy, methotrexate, ciclosporin or acitretin) and, for psoriatic arthritis, at least two disease modifying drugs (DMARDs).
- Those who have tried systemic medications but need to come off them due to side effects.
- In a person with psoriatic arthritis, there must be three or more tender joints and three or more swollen joints before biologics will be offered.

7

Phototherapy

In the human body, the two uppermost layers of skin are actually damaged when sunlight filters through them. This is because the genetic material (known as DNA) that they contain is violently bombarded by ultraviolet radiation. The normal activity of immune system cells in the skin is also undermined – and the result of both processes is ageing skin, wrinkles and even skin cancer. It is only fortunate that light – whether natural or artificial – can also destroy the cells that form psoriasis patches. Moreover, it improves blood circulation, thereby providing the body with the nutrients that it requires for healing.

Phototherapy – the use of natural or artificial light for medical purposes – can be delivered in the form of UVA or UVB radiation (UV stands for ultraviolet and the 'A' or 'B' is simply a form of classification). However, phototherapy is not suitable for everyone. For instance, some people with psoriasis are sensitive to sunlight and those with very severe psoriasis cannot tolerate further stress on the skin.

Although sunlight contains both UVA and UVB light, it is UVB light that is the main cause of sunburn, chiefly affecting the outer layers of skin. UVB also slows down the overproduction of skin cells as seen in psoriasis.

Here are more facts about UVA and UVB therapies:

- In an analysis in 2000 that compared several of the treatments for psoriasis, the highest complete clearance rate (in 86 per cent of patients) was achieved by UVB.
- When delivered as a treatment, UVB is approximately 1,000 times more powerful than UVA in causing sunburn. As a result, it can produce only a pale flush to the skin and still be effective against psoriasis. When UVA produces the same skin tone, little good has been done.

- In comparison with UVB, there is a greater risk of skin cancer, including melanoma, occurring from the use of UVA.
- UVB is normally delivered without a photosensitizing agent, unlike UVA. To be effective, UVA must be used with such an agent, usually one called psoralen – it is then known as PUVA therapy. This is then more powerful than the UVB therapies. The PUVA approach may not be easy to tolerate, but is thought to be effective in more than 85 per cent of cases.
- Some hospitals and medical centres prefer to use PUVA therapy, while others prefer to use UVB therapy. Basically, which therapy you are offered may depend on your geographical location.
- The effectiveness of phototherapy may be improved when combined with a topical treatment or a systemic agent (see Chapter 6). The addition of another agent may also speed healing.

PUVA therapy

As mentioned above, when UVA light therapy is combined with an oral medication called psoralen, it is known as PUVA therapy. Psoralen makes UVA – normally a less potent treatment than UVB – far more effective. The risk of side effects is greater, however:

- Sunburn-like photoreactions can occur, and are more severe than those that can result from UVB treatment.
- There is a small risk of developing squamous cell carcinoma in the future.[7]
- There may be an increased risk of melanoma occurring. [8]
- After a few years of PUVA therapy, unusual pigmented lesions may appear.

The drug acitretin is often combined with PUVA to improve its efficacy, particularly for pustular and erythrodermic psoriasis. Acitretin is probably the safest systemic treatment; it is also capable of shortening the PUVA treatment period and lowering the long-term risk of skin cancers.

A chemical reaction between psoralen and light, which occurs in the skin, inhibits skin cell growth and causes redness and inflammation. This damage slows down the overproduction of skin cells and reduces the formation of plaques. If you are light-sensitive or taking drugs that make you light-sensitive, protective measures will be taken on your behalf before the therapy starts.

Psoralen is taken by mouth 75–120 minutes before the commencement of the light treatment. It travels through the bloodstream to the skin where it increases the skin's sensitivity to UVA radiation. Sometimes topical preparations of psoralen are used, which may require you to bathe in a psoralen solution. You will be given special goggles to protect your eyes, then asked to stand in a light box, starting with a few seconds of exposure and going up to perhaps 20 minutes. During the treatment, you will be checked several times to ensure that you are all right.

You may need to have such treatment two or three times a week. In general, it takes about 25 treatments to achieve the best effect.

UVB therapy

Although UVB therapy can cause sunburn reactions, it is extremely safe. Because it can cause ageing of the skin in the long term, the face is protected during treatment. Another potential risk is thought to be skin cancer, but in studies over several years not one case of skin cancer occurred. If a person has already had skin cancer, however, a different treatment should probably be sought.

UVB therapy can be combined with other treatments to produce better clearance. If there is initial control of the problem, long-term remission of the disease can often be achieved.

UVB therapy is usually carried out three or four times a week as a day-treatment regimen, and patients report that they enjoy the process. UVB therapies can be broadband or narrowband, as described below.

Broadband UVB

Broadband UVB is a less potent UVB therapy that is commonly used, but it is not sufficiently effective for chronic severe psoriasis. When combined with medications, broadband UVB is usually first administered in a medical environment. Once the disease process becomes stable, the necessary equipment is given to you so you can treat yourself at home.

Before using the equipment, you will need to undress and cover any sensitive areas, starting off with a few seconds of exposure to the rays and slowly building up. It is important to be vigilant during and after the treatment, reducing the exposure time for a while if any itching or irritation occurs. Between 20 and 40 treatments may be required, at the rate of about three a week.

Coal tar, anthralin or a simple emollient such as Vaseline can increase UVB light penetration and achieve better, faster results. Great care must be taken, however, since the use of topical treatments can increase the risk of sunburn. Combining broadband UVB with oral agents such as methotrexate or oral retinoids can give very good results, but must be supervised by a doctor.

Narrowband UVB

Some experts believe that narrowband UVB should be the first option for the treatment of chronic plaque psoriasis – fewer sessions are generally required to achieve a good clearance and it is considered a very safe treatment, even for children and pregnant women. It is typical for a clearance rate of 75 per cent to occur after only 10–12 treatments.

Unfortunately, recent studies have indicated that narrowband UVB has no positive effect on the disease process itself – it merely clears the psoriasis on a very temporary basis. To date it is not really known whether it is of true value as a treatment of psoriasis.

The effectiveness of narrowband UVB can be improved by the application of topical agents such as psoralen or tazarotene. Note that narrowband UVB can never be combined with systemic medications.

Laser treatment

A variation of a device called an excimer laser is proving successful at reducing local areas of psoriasis. It delivers a precise UVB wavelength that targets specific areas of skin, sparing the healthy surrounding skin. Normally, only eight to ten sessions are required, taken twice a week; a lower dose of ultraviolet radiation is delivered than in other phototherapy treatments. A common side effect is blistering. Further studies are required to determine the long-term risks and benefits compared with other forms of phototherapy.

Tanning beds

UVB therapy can also be obtained by the use of commercial tanning beds. Such beds are available in virtually all towns in the UK and may be useful for patients who don't have easy access to a UVB treatment centre. However, tanning beds and home tanning devices are not recommended by dermatologists for the treatment of psoriasis for the following reasons:

- They are not medically supervised.
- They use both UVA and UVB, and it is not known whether the UVA tanning light is effective at clearing psoriasis or whether it is a contaminant of the UVB light.
- The ultraviolet output of different tanning beds varies widely.
- There is the same risk of side effects as with any other photo-therapy treatment, including a risk of skin cancer.

Tanning beds may be seen as an option only for someone who is unable to obtain UVB phototherapy in a medical environment.

8
Self-help

Although it's important to follow your doctor's advice and a medical treatment plan, a good deal of psoriasis care is up to you. Indeed, many people subscribe to the view that the condition can be effectively managed through a healthy lifestyle. This involves minimizing stress and eating a healthy diet, combined with plenty of rest and some sunshine. This type of long-term management strategy can be supplemented by following a solicitous self-care routine (such as discussed below). These things can't cure the condition but they can significantly improve symptoms, making damaged skin look and feel better and enabling you to get on with your life.

Self-help advice

Here are a few commonsense self-help ideas to help to minimize psoriasis flare-ups:

Take daily baths

Bathing daily in warm water – not hot – can help to soak off scales and calm inflamed skin. Add an aromatherapy oil, oiled oatmeal, Epsom salts or Dead Sea salts to the water, then soak for about 15 minutes. Spending much longer than 15 minutes in a bath can tend to dry out your skin.

As normal soap can be drying to the skin, look for mild soaps with added fats and oils. Some people find greater benefit from washing with aqueous cream or an emollient such as E45 cream.

When you get out of the bath, don't automatically rub your skin with the towel as you might if you didn't have psoriasis – rubbing only irritates it. Instead, use the towel to carefully blot or pat each section of skin. Avoid pulling the towel to and fro between your toes. Instead, you can gently pull your toes apart and pat the area with the towel.

Apply moisturizer

After patting your skin with a towel, apply moisturizer right away, while your skin is still damp – using moisturizers on damp skin is especially effective. Use a heavy, ointment-based cream to soothe and soften the skin – however, if your skin is naturally very dry, it's probably best to use oil. Oils stay on the skin longer than creams and lotions and help to stop fluids evaporating from the skin. Creams and lotions that contain alcohol should be avoided. Very dry skin responds better when moisturizer is applied several times a day.

Avoid injuring the skin

However much you are tempted to scratch or pick at your skin, it's important that you don't. It may bleed and become infected, giving psoriasis an opportunity to develop in that area. For the same reason, any other form of injury should be avoided, such as bumping yourself against a hard object, grazing yourself against something sharp or burning yourself with the iron.

Like scratching, picking at the affected areas can cause bleeding and infection. If the dryness of your skin is encouraging you to pick at it, you probably need to use larger amounts of skin-softening creams and lotions on a more regular basis.

Cover affected areas overnight

You can help yourself by applying a thick moisturizer to the affected areas of skin at night and, if possible, wrapping with cling film. In the morning, remove the cling film and take a bath or shower. This will wash away all the loosened scales.

Sunlight exposure

Many people with mild to moderate psoriasis feel that regular exposure to the sun is beneficial – and indeed, since sunlight exposure can slow down cell growth, it is likely to improve lesions. However, be careful to control the amount of sunlight you expose yourself to, because overexposure can trigger an outbreak or worsen one that is already present. Too much sunlight on the skin can also increase the risk of skin cancer, which is raised slightly already in psoriasis. If you want to sunbathe, apply sunscreen with a sun protection factor of at least 15, paying particular attention to your hands, face and ears – then try spending no longer than 20 minutes in the sun, maybe three times a week. If you feel that amount is beneficial, try spending a couple more minutes in the sun and noting its effect. Don't ever spend long periods in the sun, even if you are wearing sunscreen – and at all costs avoid getting sunburnt. You should aim for a light tan, no more.

If you are planning a holiday, consider taking it in a sunny area such as the Mediterranean or the Caribbean regions. For those who can afford it, spending several weeks at the Dead Sea in Israel has been proved to give 88 per cent clearance of the affected areas, in some cases. In this area there is a unique combination of minerals and salts from the sea together with intense but naturally filtered UVA radiation from the sun.

Some people find that direct exposure to the sun causes their psoriasis to flare up and cause irritation and pain. They should therefore always apply sunscreen with a sun protection factor of 30 or above when out in the sun and make sure that their clothes cover their arms, legs, neck and chest.

Help for the winter months

Humidity levels are generally lower in the winter months, especially in homes with forced air heating. As this tends to make the skin dry and itchy, you need to increase your use of moisturizing creams and ointments, applying heavy layers especially to areas affected by psoriasis. For the best results, apply creams and ointments after having a bath or shower while your skin is still damp.

Wear cotton clothes

In psoriasis, it is always best to wear cotton clothes next to your skin. Avoid wearing rough, synthetic materials because they can irritate psoriasis and may cause you to scratch.

Avoid known triggers

If possible, take note of the things that trigger or worsen your psoriasis and try to avoid them. Examples might be stress, injuries to the skin, infections, overexposure to the sun, stress, smoking and drinking alcohol.

Keep your fingernails short

Although some scratching may be inevitable, especially when you are asleep and free from conscious control, you will do yourself less harm if your fingernails are short.

Avoid using abrasive cleaning fluids

Abrasive cleansers, harsh detergents and household chemicals should be avoided.

Wear special gloves at night

If you scratch in your sleep or if you itch more when you are lying in bed and all is quiet, think of wearing special gloves made of Gore-Tex. The gloves can be worn over a thick moisturizing cream. They are protective, but allow your hands to 'breathe'.

Use an anti-dandruff shampoo

To control scalp psoriasis, use only anti-dandruff shampoo or products that are designed to remove scales (keratolytics), that counter inflammatory effects and that generally calm the skin.

Maintain a healthy weight

Maintaining a healthy weight is important to overall health. The best way to increase nutrients whilst limiting your calories is to eat more fruit, vegetables and whole grains. Drinking plenty of water is also recommended.

Pace yourself

Living with an uncomfortable disorder with possible social and psychological implications can leave you feeling drained. Moreover, you are more likely than many other people to be anaemic, so you should take care not to overdo it. Don't stop being active, just learn to listen to your body and rest before you become tired. Dividing exercise sessions and work activities into small segments can be enormously helpful, as can finding the time to relax at regular intervals throughout the day.

Educate yourself

Finding out as much as possible about psoriasis will make it appear far less daunting. It can also help you to understand the possible triggers so that you are more able to prevent flare-ups. Educating your family and friends can help them to understand your efforts in dealing with the condition and may encourage their support.

Have a strong support network

The support of your doctor, family and friends can make a great difference to how you cope with a chronic disorder such as psoriasis. We all know that having someone to talk to at a difficult time can be an enormous boost, enabling you to feel less helpless and alone. Knowing we are cared about also makes us more likely to take good care of ourselves. Stress levels are lowered, too, when we know we are supported.

Join a psoriasis support group

People who don't have too many family and friends – or who are concerned about burdening loved ones – can find that attending a local support group with people who know what you're going through makes them feel less emotionally isolated. It's usually comforting to share your experiences and struggles and to speak to people who have undergone similar things. Swapping practical information and advice can also be a great help.

There are now psoriasis support groups in most areas, with further groups being set up. If you are interested in joining one, ask your doctor for information. Support groups don't suit everyone, however.

Exercise

If possible, carrying out a daily exercise routine, or getting involved in recreational activities such as badminton, swimming or tennis, can help in the following ways:

- It slows down bone loss, increases flexibility, strengthens the muscles that stabilize the joints, reduces morning stiffness and maintains mobility – these results are often particularly beneficial to people with psoriatic arthritis; indeed, many people with psoriatic arthritis who take regular exercise say that they experience less pain and fatigue.

- It reduces your levels of stress – one of the exacerbating factors in psoriasis.
- It stimulates the lymph glands which operate as a drainage system to rid the body of harmful toxins. The flow of lymph from the lymph glands is largely dependent upon muscular movement.
- It floods your body with endorphins – endorphins being natural 'feel-good' chemicals that give you a 'lift' and a sense of wellbeing.
- It helps to control your weight.

You are the best judge of how much exercise you can do. Just bear in mind that an appropriate level of activity should make you feel the same or better afterwards – never worse. Gradually introduce new activities and heed the warning signs so you don't overdo things. If you experience new or increased pain later in the day or fatigue the next day, you've done too much!

People with psoriatic arthritis may need physiotherapy to help to improve joint mobility and function. During physiotherapy splints may be used to hold the joints in place and reduce pain and inflammation. Occupational therapy may also be offered to someone with psoriatic arthritis. This can help you to function far more effectively in the home and in leisure time.

It is best to avoid contact sports such as football and rugby. Such sports can cause many bumps and scrapes which will only worsen your psoriasis.

Self-help for specific areas

Specific areas such as skin folds, the mouth and the genitals often fall victim to psoriasis. However, improvements can come from following a particular routine, as described below. When hydrocortisone cream is recommended, as it is in a few cases, take care not to use it for prolonged periods since this can permanently thin the skin.

Always use medications as directed.

Psoriasis in skin folds

As a condition called intertrigo – a superficial fungal and bacterial infection – can closely mimic psoriasis in folds of the skin, your doctor needs first of all to determine what exactly the problem is. It isn't helped at all by the two conditions often being present at the same time, in which case they must be treated simultaneously. You can do this by purchasing an over-the-counter anti-inflammatory cream such as hydrocortisone cream for twice-daily application in a very thin layer. Add a thin layer of an over-the-counter antifungal cream, mix it with the anti-inflammatory, then cover with a thin layer of a good moisturizing cream.

Regularly soaking in a salt or tar bath will also provide relief from itching and help to improve the condition. If this treatment regime fails to work, seek help from your doctor.

Facial psoriasis

The most common areas for facial psoriasis are the forehead and upper lip. Facial psoriasis can resemble seborrhoeic dermatitis (including dandruff) and so may be treated unsatisfactorily. You can ease facial psoriasis by applying a moisturizer or petroleum jelly at regular intervals. If this doesn't help, try an over-the-counter hydrocortisone cream, applied twice daily. On top of this, use a good moisturizer or petroleum jelly.

It may also be helpful to spend 15–20 minutes in direct sunlight each day, if at all possible. Use a high-factor sun protection cream to ensure that you don't burn. Take care to keep the cream away from your eyes.

Psoriasis around the eyes

Psoriasis in the area of the eyes is particularly nasty. If the eyelid is affected, use an eyebath to apply a solution of lukewarm tap water and baby shampoo twice daily. Next use a face cloth to rub the eyelid gently in order to remove excess scale. Rather than using hydrocortisone cream, a good moisturizer should then be applied.

If the inner lining of the eye is affected, this very sensitive area should receive special treatment and you should seek the help of your optician.

Psoriasis in the mouth

It is possible for psoriasis to arise on the tongue or the mucous membranes of the mouth or lips. The best self-treatment is good dental hygiene twice daily, including rinsing out the mouth with a saline solution. If the lips are affected, try applying an over-the-counter hydrocortisone cream. See your doctor if these recommendations fail.

Psoriasis in the ears

Great care should be taken when creams are used in the delicate area of the inside of the ears. It is probably best to use an earwax removal kit, which is available from your local pharmacy. Follow the instructions very carefully, to keep the area lubricated and to control scaling, and then apply a thin layer of mineral oil and warm water to the ear canal. In severe cases, try applying over-the-counter hydrocortisone cream twice daily. If such self-treatments fail, seek your doctor's help.

Psoriasis on the hands and feet

In psoriasis, it is common to have plaques on your hands and feet. As cracking and infection can easily occur in these areas, the treatment regimen is more aggressive and must be carried out twice daily.

The thickness and scaling of the skin can be helped by soaking your hands and feet in a tar or salt bath for 20–30 minutes at least once a day. Afterwards, you should use a skin file or pumice stone to rub off the loose skin gently. Next apply a topical cortisone cream – any large cracks should be very carefully closed with Superglue or a skin-bonding glue. If this is your last treatment of the day and you are going to bed, it will also be helpful to bind your hands and feet in cellophane wrap, avoiding pulling too tightly. Another perhaps more acceptable alternative is to use damp cotton gloves or socks, keeping them on for at least two hours.

Genital psoriasis

Unfortunately, genital psoriasis is common and may even be present in isolation. In this area the skin is naturally thin and sensitive, and psoriasis tends to appear as non-scaly, red plaques, which may itch or hurt.

As this area is very sensitive, it should initially be treated in the same way as the scalp – when bathing apply a medicated shampoo, leaving it on for five or ten minutes. A mild cortisone cream, such as over-the-counter hydrocortisone cream, may then be applied twice daily. To tackle itchiness, soak in a tar or salt bath twice a day for 20–30 minutes. Anti-itch creams could be liberally applied throughout the day, too.

You should also find relief from wearing loose-fitting undergarments, preferably made from breathable fabrics such as cotton. Avoid feminine hygiene products, since they often contain latex, which has been known to aggravate psoriasis. Steer clear of permanent press clothing, too, since it contains formaldehyde, which may exacerbate the condition.

Herbal remedies

Many people are of the opinion that herbs and other dietary supplements are safer than chemical drugs because they are 'natural'. However, 'natural' doesn't automatically mean safe, one reason being that herbal remedies can interfere with prescription drugs. Moreover, their quality, safety and effectiveness are not regulated by a governing body. In fact, serious side effects can occur if they are not taken with care. You should therefore always inform your doctor of any herbal remedies and dietary supplements that you are taking, and you should follow the dosage instructions on the label very carefully.

In this section some of the herbal remedies recognized as being useful in treating psoriasis are discussed. If you are at all unsure of how to prepare and use them, don't hesitate to consult an experienced herbalist, who will not only ensure that you are obtaining the most suitable remedies but will also offer step-by-step guidance. A trained herbalist will be able to prescribe more potent remedies that are not on general sale, too.

The herbs mentioned below are available from most health-food shops, usually as dried herbs, tablets or tincture.

Evening primrose oil

Although there are many anecdotal reports of evening primrose oil improving psoriasis, studies have not revealed a significant effect. If you wish to try it, follow the label dosage instructions.

Evening primrose oil can also be used as a topical treatment for the skin. No studies have been conducted into the effects of this oil on psoriasis, but when tested on people with eczema there was significant reduction in symptoms and the overall severity of the condition. It can therefore be assumed that it will be of benefit in treating psoriasis, too. There have been no reports of side effects with evening primrose oil, and its safety for topical use has never been in doubt.

Oats

Oat extracts have been used for centuries in soothing topical preparations, and today they are found in many skin care products around the world. Oat plant derivatives are capable of easing dry, itchy skin conditions and many bath products incorporate colloidal oatmeal into their products as the active ingredient.

Here is an oatmeal recipe for use in the bath:

1 cup oats
¼ cup dried milk powder
2 tbsp apricot kernel oil (optional)

Pulverize the oats and dried milk powder in a food blender, then gradually add the apricot kernel oil. Place the mixture in a cotton bag, sock or handkerchief and place in the bath while it's being filled. Squeeze out the mixture while you are soaking in the bath.

Tea tree oil

Tea tree oil is produced by a native Australian species of tea tree (*Melaleuca alternifolia*) and is known for its antiseptic and antibacterial properties. Traditionally used for colds, toothaches, headaches, sore muscles and skin disorders, today it is the active ingredient in many creams, lotions, shampoos and soaps. Some people swear by it for the treatment of scalp psoriasis, and it can also be applied to other areas of skin. As no one knows what strength of tea tree oil is safe and effective, use it with care. If irritation occurs, stop using it straightaway. Tea tree oil is for topical use only – indeed, it is toxic if ingested.

Apple cider vinegar

Apple cider vinegar – commonly known as cider vinegar – has long been used as a soothing, disinfecting agent. It can be applied directly to the skin, mixed into a moisturizer or added to the bath. You can even soak your fingernails and toenails in it. Use cotton wool balls or pads when applying to the skin.

Aloe

Aloe, a member of the lily family, has been used for centuries in the treatment of burns and minor wounds. Nowadays aloe gel is often added to cosmetics, sun creams and skin care creams and ointments. There are many anecdotal tales of its effectiveness in soothing skin irritations but as yet no positive proof in the form of studies. However, aloe vera gel is undeniably very soothing and calming, so I wouldn't discourage its use.

Oil of oregano

Oregano – a herb commonly used in baking and cooking – has antibacterial and antifungal properties and as such may be helpful in treating certain of the infections that may come with psoriasis. There are many reports of oregano oil, taken orally or used topically, helping psoriasis. It should be used with caution, however, since it can cause allergic contact dermatitis when applied to the skin.

Milk thistle

The activation of T cells (see page 44) has been shown to be inhibited by the use of milk thistle products, which reduces skin cell overgrowth. Milk thistle is considered a safe herb, but in rare cases it can cause a brief gastrointestinal upset or mild allergic reaction.

Note that milk thistle should not be taken if you are also taking antipsychotic drugs or male hormones.

Shark cartilage

A range of studies have shown that shark cartilage extract prevents the formation of new blood vessels – and new blood vessel growth is known to play a role in the development and exacerbation of psoriasis lesions. As shark cartilage extract can also counter the inflammatory process, it is believed to be useful for treating psoriasis. Interestingly, clinical studies into the effects of shark cartilage extract on psoriasis are currently under way.

This supplement is taken in pill form and often referred to as AE941. The known side effects include brief nausea and skin rashes.

Turmeric

A main component of curry powder, turmeric has long been used in Chinese medicine to relieve the inflammation and pain associated with arthritic conditions. It can also be of benefit for the inflammation found in psoriasis. If you have gallstones or bile duct problems this spice should be avoided.

Capsaicin

Capsaicin ointment contains the active ingredient in hot chilli peppers and, when applied to the skin, can ease the torment of itching. Gloves should be worn to handle the ointment and to apply it to affected areas, three or four times daily. There is an initial burning sensation but this soon dies down and should diminish with use.

9

Psoriasis and nutrition

It is unfortunate that, to date, very little research into psoriasis and diet has taken place. Of course there are many claims about the beneficial effects of certain foods and types of diets on psoriasis, but whether any of these claims will ever be proved is anyone's guess. We shouldn't forget that we are all very different and what appears to be a wonderful aid for one person will not necessarily be of any help to another. Moreover, diets that restrict a particular food group can never be beneficial in the long term – in fact, they can be downright damaging. We need to eat a balanced diet comprising all food groups.

However, eliminating the one or two food substances that you know from experience will cause more itching is a different matter entirely, and you should be ever vigilant for a food (or drink) that causes a flare-up of symptoms or some other problem. Cutting it out of your diet can make a real difference to your life.

Until scientists tell us differently (if that day ever comes), it is generally accepted that the first step, diet-wise, in reducing the severity of psoriasis is to drink lots of water – about two litres a day. The second step is to eat a healthy balanced diet.

Our diet in Western societies

Nowadays, the average Western diet is very poor. It is estimated that we eat approximately 17 per cent of our daily calories as processed foods, 18 per cent as saturated fats, 18 per cent as sugar and 3–10 per cent as alcoholic beverages. When you add this up, more than half our foods are high in calories and low in nutrients. So it is little wonder that over time many of us develop chronic health problems.

Nutritious food is actually one of the finest medications we can put into our bodies, and one of the best means of influencing health. Indeed, not only does food keep us alive, it also has the ability to repair and regenerate our bodily tissues.

Today, because of chemical pesticides, food additives, preservatives and so on, we constantly ingest low levels of toxicity, which has given rise to an array of immunity disorders. Psoriasis is one such disorder.

Why good nutrition?

Nutritionists believe that eating a healthy balanced diet and taking regular exercise can diminish the severity of psoriasis. It may also help to:

- build resistance to stress;
- increase physical stamina;
- increase resistance to disease;
- encourage greater emotional stability.

Recommendations for psoriasis

Our bodies need a *wide variety* of foods and food combinations. This helps to ensure that we are ingesting a wide range of essential vitamins, minerals and fatty acids. To eat the same foods repeatedly means missing out on many important building blocks of life, for certain foods build and regenerate only certain parts of the body. A restricted diet also increases the risk of developing immune system disorders such as psoriasis.

Because the majority of our foodstuffs are grown in a chemical environment, they are low in nutrients and high in toxicity. It is advisable, therefore, to purchase organically grown produce and to look for foods without added chemicals (colourings, flavourings and preservatives).

Here are a few guidelines for improving your diet:

- Eat three or four small meals a day, with snacks in between.
- Never go more than three hours without eating something, which means you should never go hungry.
- Don't skip breakfast. After fasting during the night, the body needs glucose. When nourishment is withheld, brain function is

diminished. Studies have shown that children who eat breakfast perform better at school than those who have not eaten.

- Avoid missing a meal. When we allow ourselves to become very hungry, sugary, high-fat foods become more tempting.
- Don't overeat – not even healthy foods.
- Ensure that your snacks are nutritious and readily available. Examples are raw fruits and vegetables, fruit and vegetable juices, dried fruit, unsalted uncoated nuts, and a variety of seeds and rye crispbreads. These should not spoil your appetite for an upcoming meal. Obviously, if you suffer from a nut allergy, leave nuts alone.
- If you are counting calories, it's unhealthy to continue restricting them once you have reached your ideal weight. If you are unsure of how to maintain your ideal weight, just follow the healthy balanced diet described in the next few pages.

Foods to eat

The following is a discussion of the foods that make up a healthy balanced diet.

Fruit and vegetables

Fruit and vegetables are rich in vitamin C and other important vitamins and minerals. Try to eat as many as you can, selecting locally grown, organic fruit and vegetables that are in season – these have the highest nutrient content and the greatest enzyme activity. Enzymes are to our body what spark plugs are to the car engine. Without the 'sparks', the body doesn't work properly. Organically grown fruit and vegetables may not look as perfect as those that are processed, but they *are* superior – processed foods are devitalized of their 'sparks'.

Try to eat as fresh and as raw as possible – make a variety of salads and try to eat one every day. When you do cook vegetables, cook them in the minimum of unsalted (or lightly salted) water for the minimum length of time. Lightly steaming and stir-frying are healthy alternatives. Scrub rather than peel your vegetables.

Grapes contain resveratrol, a plant-derived non-steroidal compound that works to block inflammation – and inflammation is a fundamental problem for people with psoriasis. It is a good idea, then, to snack on grapes as often as you can. You could even add them to your salads. Remember to wash them first to remove any chemical residue.

For many years, professional coaches have encouraged their athletes to eat pineapple to help heal sports injuries. Pineapple contains a key enzyme called bromelain that also helps to reduce inflammation.

Legumes (peas and beans)

Legumes are high in protein and usually inexpensive. The soya bean is a complete protein, and there are many soya bean products, including soya milk, tofu, tempeh and miso. Tofu, for example, is very versatile and can be used in both savoury and sweet dishes.

Seeds

Sunflower, sesame, hemp and pumpkin seeds contain a wonderful combination of nutrients – all necessary to start a new plant and important to good health for us. They can be eaten as they are as a snack, sprinkled on to salads and cereals or used in baking. For more flavour they can be lightly roasted and coated with organic soy sauce.

Nuts

Nuts, too, are an intrinsic part of any healthy diet. All nuts contain vital nutrients, but almonds, cashews, walnuts, Brazil nuts and pecan nuts offer the greatest array. Eat a wide assortment as snacks, with cereal and in baking.

Grains

Whole grains and wholemeal flours provide us with the complex unrefined carbohydrates our bodies require – and again organic is best. Aim to consume a variety of grains, including oats, rye, barley (generally available as pearl barley), corn, buckwheat, brown rice and mixed grains. Oats are highly recommended, too, because they help to stabilize blood sugar levels.

Bread and other commercial grain products that are enriched with folic acid are recommended for people with psoriasis.

Fish

Try to eat plenty of fish, especially oily fish such as sardines, tuna, mackerel, trout, salmon, herring, pilchards and kippers. The omega-3 fatty acids that are found in such fish have anti-inflammatory properties that may be of benefit in treating psoriasis.

Cut down on red meat as much as possible. When you do eat red meat, make sure it is no larger or thicker than the palm of your hand.

Garlic, onions, ginger and cayenne pepper

Garlic, onions, ginger and cayenne pepper are all part of a healthy balanced diet.

Reducing salt

Although our bodies need a certain amount of the sodium that we obtain from salt, a high intake can be harmful in many ways. High blood pressure and heart disease are just two of the conditions that are linked to high salt consumption.

Salt as a preservative

Owing to its ability to inhibit the growth of harmful micro-organisms, high levels of salt are added as a preservative to most processed and pre-packaged foods. For example, one tin of soup contains more salt (sodium) than the recommended daily allowance for an adult. Large amounts of salt are also added to most breakfast cereals, except for shredded wheat products. It is recommended, therefore, that you limit your intake of salt in the following ways:

- Reduce your consumption of processed and pre-packaged foods.
- When you must buy processed and pre-packaged foods, look for 'low-salt' or 'sodium-free' on the label.
- Use only a very small amount of sea salt or rock salt in baking and cooking.
- Try to avoid sprinkling any type of salt over your meals.

Reducing your salt intake very gradually is the best way to retrain your palate.

Reducing stimulants

One of the main reasons we crave stimulants such as caffeine, cigarettes and products containing white refined sugar is high levels of stress. When we are stressed our bodies demand a boost of energy – a 'lift'. However, the lift we obtain from stimulants is short-lived, unlike the damage it can cause to our bodies.

Cutting out stimulants can have the following benefits:

- It can significantly raise energy levels.
- It can reduce anxiety.
- It can improve the health of our nerve cells.

If you find you are unable to eliminate completely stimulants from your diet, reduce them as much as possible – it *will* make a difference.

Sugar

You may be surprised to hear that sugar consumption has been linked with many disorders, from diabetes to heart disease and cancer. However, we do need a certain amount of sugar for conversion to energy. But we can actually obtain all the sugar that we need from fruit and from complex (unrefined) carbohydrates (in grains, lentils and so on), which convert into sugar in the body as nature intended.

If you really need to sweeten your food and drinks, alternatives to refined white sugar include raw honey, barley malt and fruit juice sweetener (fructose). Muscovado sugar and demerara sugar (both of which are also referred to as 'soft brown sugar') are formed during the early stages of the sugar refining process and so contain more nutrients than refined white sugar. The above-mentioned may all be used in cooking and baking.

Artificial sweeteners

Refined sugar and simple carbohydrates are best avoided, so can they be replaced by a sugar substitute such as aspartame? The short answer is no, not if you really want to be healthy. Aspartame is an excitatory neurotransmitter (nerve transmitter) that causes nerve cells to fire excessively.

Many people consume food and drinks containing aspartame in an attempt to lose weight. However, this artificial sweetener creates a craving for carbohydrates, which only causes weight gain. When people stop using aspartame – in diet sodas, for example – they generally lose weight.

The unrefined sugars found naturally in fruit and vegetables are safe and nutritious. They also take longer to digest, which avoids a sugar rush to the bloodstream and thus excessive production of insulin. Fortunately, there are natural sweeteners such as stevia and xylitol that are perfectly safe and available from health food shops.

Fats and oils

There are two types of fat – saturated and unsaturated. The two distinct types are described below:

Saturated fat

Saturated fat and trans-fatty acids have a negative effect on the circulatory system. They increase blood levels of bad cholesterol, decrease levels of good cholesterol and can lead to atherosclerosis – a disease of the arteries characterized by deposits of fatty material on the artery walls. Atherosclerosis in turn can lead to heart disease and stroke because it impedes normal blood flow through the arteries. Saturated fat comes mainly from animal sources and is generally solid at room temperature.

Note that although margarine was, for many years, believed to be a healthier choice over butter, nutritionists have now revised their opinion, for some of the fats in the margarine hydrogenation process are changed into trans-fatty acids, which the body metabolizes as if they were saturated fatty acids – the same as butter. Butter is a valuable source of oils and vitamin A, but should be used very sparingly. Margarine, on the other hand, is an artificial product containing many additives.

Unsaturated fat

Also called polyunsaturated or monounsaturated fat, unsaturated fat has a protective effect on the heart and other organs. Omega-3 and omega-6 oils occur naturally in oily fish (such as mackerel, herring, sardines and tuna), nuts and seeds, and are usually liquid at room temperature. It is recommended that we all eat oily fish at least three times a week and cold-pressed oil (olive, rapeseed, safflower and sunflower oil) daily, in dressings and in cooking. Olive oil is better suited to cooking than other oils because it suffers less damage from heat.

Eggs

You're no doubt aware that eggs are high in cholesterol, a type of fat. However, they also contain lecithin, which is a superb biological detergent capable of breaking down fats so they can be utilized by the body. Lecithin also prevents the accumulation of too many acid or alkaline substances in the blood and encourages the transport of nutrients through the cell walls. Eggs should be soft-boiled or poached as a hard yolk will bind the lecithin, rendering it useless as a fat-detergent.

It is recommended that you eat two or three eggs a week.

Retraining your palate

In comparison with the average Western diet, which has (through the addition of chemical flavourings, saturated fat, sugar, salt and so on) evolved largely to please the taste buds, a healthy diet is based on foods in their more natural form. It is essential, therefore, that you should *slowly* retrain your palate to accept different tastes. For this reason, it is advisable to cut back gradually on the amounts of sugar, salt and saturated fat that you consume. It takes only 28 days of eating a food regularly for it to become a habit.

Alcohol

Research has shown very clearly that people who drink a lot of alcohol have a greater chance of developing psoriasis than those who don't. The reasons for that aren't yet evident, however. Even so, a great many studies into the effects of alcohol intake on psoriasis have been carried out. Here are their general conclusions:

- High alcohol intake is one of the risk factors for psoriasis.
- Some people are heavy drinkers before they develop psoriasis.
- Of the people with psoriasis who were studied, the heavy drinkers were more likely to be men than women.
- Men with psoriasis drink more than men without.
- The incidence of psoriasis is greater among alcoholics than among those who don't drink to excess. Those who abstain from drinking alcohol are the least likely of all to develop psoriasis.
- Heavy drinking is a typical trigger of a psoriasis flare-up.
- Heavy drinking can prevent an important medication from working.
- Many people use alcohol to cope with the emotional aspects of psoriasis such as the unattractive appearance of their skin.

If you drink a lot of alcohol, it's strongly advised that you limit your intake to, at most, the level considered 'safe'. In the UK, it is considered that the weekly safe limit for women is no more than 14 units, and for men it is a maximum of 21 units:

- Half a pint of normal strength beer, lager or cider equals one unit.
- A small (100 ml) glass of wine equals one unit.
- A large (175 ml) glass of wine equals approximately two units.
- A single (25 ml) measure of spirits equals one unit.
- A 275 ml bottle of alcopop (5.5%/volume) equals 1.5 units.

If you are taking a systemic medication such as methotrexate, it's strongly recommended that you don't drink alcohol at all. (See Chapter 6 for details of systemic medications.)

Smoking

Smoking is not just a factor in the onset of psoriasis, it is liable to make the disease significantly worse. There are thousands of different compounds in cigarette smoke, which make it difficult to assess how the smoke might affect a person on a biological level. However, nicotine, for instance, is believed to affect cell growth, impede immune system function and encourage inflammation of the skin.

There have been hundreds of studies into the link between smoking and psoriasis. Here are their general conclusions:

- There is a far higher incidence of psoriasis in people who smoke than in non-smokers. Indeed, approximately one in five cases appears to be related to smoking.
- The number of cigarettes (or cigars) smoked per day relates to the risk of getting psoriasis – the more smoked, the higher the risk.
- There is a very strong link between smoking and a type of pustular psoriasis called palmoplantar pustulosis.
- People with psoriasis are more likely to be obese and to smoke than people who don't have psoriasis. However, where smoking affects the onset of psoriasis, obesity does not.
- Many people use smoking to cope with the emotional twists and turns of psoriasis.

Information on dietary supplements

Until recently, there were varied opinions regarding dietary supplements for the treatment of psoriasis. For instance, some recommended vitamins A, D and E, whereas others disputed their safety. Researchers have now made the situation a little clearer, stating that vitamin D is not beneficial when taken in the normal daily allowance as recommended by the European Union, but that vitamin A may be useful. As yet there is no decisive opinion on the benefits of vitamin E, when taken as fish oil. The situation is explained in greater detail below.

Vitamin A (beta-carotene)

Researchers have found that using vitamin A for psoriasis can help skin cells to grow to maturity before shedding. It can also help to prevent infection, increase blood flow to the skin, counteract inflammation and provide protection from sunburn. Severe psoriasis can be treated by a potent form of vitamin A called etretinate.

Food sources of vitamin A include liver, fish oils, egg yolk, yellow and orange fruits and vegetables such as carrots, sweet potatoes, apricots, cantaloupe, papaya, pumpkin, melon and mango. Beta-carotene can also be found in dark leafy vegetables such as spinach, broccoli, cabbage and parsley.

Fish oil supplements

A range of studies into the effects of fish oil supplementation in the treatment of psoriasis have shown widely differing results, and the benefit, if any, is still not clear. However, there are many anecdotal reports of improvements in itching and scales. As vitamins A and D are present in fish oil, there is also the concern that fish oil supplementation – particularly cod liver oil – can cause excessive levels of these vitamins. Blood clotting can occur if high doses of fish oils are taken.

If you want to try using fish oil supplementation, it is advisable to speak to your doctor first.

10

Emotional help

'The heartbreak of psoriasis' is a phrase that originated from a 1960s advertising campaign for a coal tar-based hair product. The phrase is still used today in newspapers and magazines that either discuss the condition or advertise psoriasis treatments. Unfortunately, the phrase also often reflects the tendency for advertisers to dramatize and embellish certain features of the condition for financial gain. Ironically, though, it is very close to the truth. It describes in a nut-shell the emotional impact of the condition – a life-long disorder that is at the same time uncomfortable and unattractive and has numerous psychological and social ramifications.

The mind and body are integrally linked, which means that your beliefs about yourself and your psoriasis can have a dramatic influence on your health. When you have good self-esteem, are generally optimistic and believe you are in control of your illness, it becomes much easier to cope. It also enables you to function more effectively.

Quality of life

Quality of life is affected by all forms of psoriasis, whether mild or severe. It's common to have itching, soreness and even pain – for example, a small act like making a cup of tea can really hurt for people with severe psoriasis. However, for the majority, it's the appearance of their skin that can be very distressing and lead to the wearing of odd clothing to cover it. It can even result in some people confining themselves indoors.

For many people, awareness of their psoriasis prevents them from enjoying or even participating in their preferred leisure-time activities, and can even make it difficult to perform efficiently at work. Both of these cause frustration, but it is the failure to perform well at work that perhaps has the greatest impact, for it can lead to a drop in self-esteem, the disdain of higher management and often derision from fellow workers who may feel you are no longer pulling your weight. According to the National Psoriasis Foundation in the USA, 26 per cent of people with moderate to severe psoriasis have had to change or even stop doing the things they would normally do in a day.

When quality of life is affected, as it is in psoriasis, the result is significant stress. It is known that people with psoriasis experience more depression, anxiety and general anger than the norm, and unfortunately many try to cope by smoking tobacco or trying to blot out the negative feelings by drinking too much alcohol. And as we have seen, smoking and drinking can not only bring on a flare-up, they can significantly worsen the disease in the long term.

Self-confidence

Psoriasis can affect self-confidence so badly that it darkens almost every aspect of a person's life. As well as leisure and work activities, it impinges on social interactions, often making the person feel like an outcast. Psoriasis can also cause love-life problems, in both a physical and psychological way.

In surveys, people aged 18–24 years experienced the most dramatic blows to their self-confidence. People with visible psoriasis – on their face, scalp or hands – were the most affected. Surveys have also shown that single people and women experience the most psychological distress – single people because they have no 'other half' to help them to feel protected and reassured, and women because they tend to be far more wrapped up in what they look like than men.

Psoriasis and the general public

The perception of being misunderstood by the public is a major problem for people with psoriasis – indeed, many report feeling like social outcasts. Most of all, they fear that psoriasis is seen as contagious and that the sight of it engenders disgust.

In a recent omnibus survey of 1,000 adults without psoriasis, the vast majority of respondents (88 per cent) had heard of psoriasis and almost half actually knew someone who had the condition. Most were unaware of how common it is, but a high 86 per cent realized that it is not contagious. Moreover, 52 per cent were aware that psoriasis is more emotionally troublesome than physically disabling.

These results were a real surprise to psoriasis associations. Of course, it's horrible to have people stare at you, but we all seem to do it when faced with something that's different than the norm. Often when people look, they actually feel compassion for the other person – I know I do when my eyes are drawn for a split second to someone who's scarred or disabled in some way.

Psoriasis and your closest relationship(s)

Psoriasis is notorious for exerting strain on relationships, which in turn erodes self-confidence and causes chronic anxiety. In a romantic relationship it's natural to want the other person to see you as attractive – this enables you to feel sexy and desirable. But when psoriasis puts its stain on your skin, you may feel unattractive and wonder how anyone could truly desire you – you need to feel desirable in yourself before you can believe that another person finds you desirable. Therefore you may be beset with worries that the other person is secretly repelled and would really prefer to be with someone else, someone with normal skin. In some cases, no amount of attempted reassurance from the other person has any effect and the relationship is only a shadow of what it should be.

Many people with psoriasis are so embarrassed about their appearance that they will only get undressed or will only agree to be intimate with the lights out. This, too, can prevent them from getting emotionally close, or can cause a loving relationship to grow more distant.

I can only say that your partner is unlikely to have chosen you solely because of your looks. If so, there's a good chance he or she would go off you anyway as the years pass and you change with age (as we all do). I agree that looks are important in the early days of a relationship – some boyfriends or girlfriends may indeed be put off by your psoriasis and decide that you aren't the right one for them. But neither is he or she the right one for you! Relationships that last owe far more to shared interests and attractiveness of personality than attractiveness of physical looks, and those that start out with looks as the main draw might well fall by the wayside somewhere down the line.

On the other hand, if you are nice-looking and have a good or average body, these things don't mysteriously become invisible so that all that can be seen is your psoriasis. A partner or prospective partner who truly likes or loves and respects you will be able to see through the marks on your skin to your face and body, and of course beneath those to the inner person with all of your strengths and failings. Indeed, such a person might say that your psoriasis is part of you and that they like or love you with it and would not like or love you more without it.

If your partner or prospective partner attempts to reassure you that the appearance of your skin is not important, you need to believe that. For the strength and endurance of your relationship, it's important that you do.

Where psoriasis is in effect the third party in the relationship, many couples benefit greatly from counselling. Don't be afraid to speak to your doctor about this.

Pain during intimacy

The itching and general discomfort and pain of psoriasis often stretches to the genital areas, which of course affects sexual relations. Your best course of action here is to follow the self-care advice on page 40. If this doesn't help, ask your doctor. There may be something else you can do to ease the discomfort.

If your partner indicates that he or she would like sexual relations, but you are experiencing a flare-up of symptoms in the genital area, you must explain that you would love to but really can't. A decent, caring partner will understand and wait until you feel more up to it.

Family interactions

It is fortunate that, according to surveys, most people with psoriasis feel that their family understands what they are going through and so are supportive. Maybe, in many cases, it's easier to understand the condition because other family members may have it.

Passing on the condition

If a parent has a son or daughter with psoriasis, there tend to be a lot of guilty feelings about having 'passed it on'. Would-be parents with psoriasis usually worry that they will pass it on to their children. As mentioned earlier, when both parents have psoriasis, their children have a 50–75 per cent chance of developing the condition, whereas if only one parent is affected, the children have a 25 per cent chance of developing it. However, I hope that reading this book gives you some helpful ideas on dealing with psoriasis should it affect a child.

Social interactions

Public interaction is often avoided by people with psoriasis. When they do have to go to a meeting, a wedding or on holiday, for example, they may dress to hide their condition with long sleeves and long trousers or a long skirt, yet still manage to feel acutely aware of any remaining visible signs of the disease. Their odd clothing then makes them feel like outcasts – particularly if it's summer weather, or they are on holiday.

Surveys have shown that people who cover large areas of their bodies – usually those with more extensive psoriasis – experience more negative feelings and lower self-esteem than those who do not.

Psoriasis and school or work

When you have psoriasis, school or work can be a problem in many ways. For a start, young people can be particularly embarrassed – in early life looks count a lot. Younger children have a nasty habit of teasing anyone who doesn't fit in with the norm appearance-wise, and this can cause scars that linger well into adulthood. Teenagers also hate looking different from their peers in any way. Indeed they want very much to look good so that they fit in with the 'popular crowd', and most of all they are keen to appear desirable to the opposite sex. They may experience acute embarrassment when they have to show their bodies, such as during gym lessons or at the swimming baths. Summer can be a problem, too, giving them the dilemma of either wearing fashionable shorts, short skirts and short sleeves – thus displaying their psoriasis for all the world to see – or covering up with old-fashioned clothing that makes them look ridiculous, in their eyes.

Psoriasis can also cause physical problems at school and at work, particularly if you have psoriatic arthritis and your wrist movements are limited, or psoriasis of the hands, the skin of which is liable to crack and bleed at the least bit of physical stress. Hence, writing and drawing may be a problem at school. Obviously, problems at work depend on what exactly your job is and which form of psoriasis you have. Jobs requiring physical exertion such as fire-fighting, plumbing and construction work may be hampered by psoriasis, as may jobs requiring manual dexterity, such as hairdressing, using a computer, cake decorating and so on. Changing your job for one that is physically easier for you is not always an option either, but if it is I would say do it.

Understanding negative emotions

Psoriasis is capable of generating high levels of stress. These come not only from the negative feelings your appearance may engender and the discomfort and difficulty of functioning in daily life, but also from the sense of hopelessness you may feel in terms of a cure for the condition. Stress in itself can lead to further problems such as depression and so on, and for that reason it is important that it is reduced as much as possible.

The section that follows is aimed at helping you to understand some of the emotions you may be experiencing – and understanding them means taking a great step toward lowering your levels of stress.

I feel so vulnerable!

Vulnerability is a natural human condition. We all need people to love us; we all crave the affirmation of others. To a large extent we are all dependent upon others, measuring their responses in order to reassure ourselves that we are worthwhile human beings, that we are indeed loveable. When we have a chronic condition that makes us feel unattractive, we believe we have little to offer the people around us – therefore we fear we are no longer loveable.

Feelings of vulnerability will always be present in chronic disease – whether or not it affects our appearance – but we can defeat the worst of them by looking less to outsiders for affirmation. We all have inner strengths and particular talents, many of which we may be unaware of. Yet if we waited for others to point them out we would be likely to be waiting for ever!

Your particular forte may be in planning and organizing, or in problem solving, or in handling finances – not necessarily out of the family setting. You may be an authority on steam engines, an inspired cook, a good listener, a talented artist, an excellent singer, a diligent student, a competent driver . . . Please do not underestimate yourself!

I feel so guilty!

Feelings of guilt are common in chronic disease. It is natural to want to lay the blame at someone's door, and many of us imagine we ourselves must have done something very wrong to deserve such retribution. But blaming either ourselves or others is pointless. Life is a lottery. Some people are rich, some poor; some clever, some not so clever; some develop a life-long health condition, some remain healthy. That's just the way it is.

Flare-ups are a perpetual threat in psoriasis. Although they can result from 'outside' influences such as a fall, a burn, a family crisis and so on, it is likely that something you chose to do exacerbated the symptoms – such as drinking heavily on a night out. And so you feel guilty. Viewing a flare-up as a learning experience may be of some consolation, as long as you really do learn from it!

I feel so afraid!

It's natural to feel afraid when you have a disorder for which there is, as yet, no cure. Fears tend to be centred around the future, and what is going to happen. You are afraid your physical and emotional problems will harm your relationships; afraid that your psoriasis will become much worse; afraid you'll have to give up your job, afraid of the long-term effects of medication . . . The list is endless.

Chronic conditions exert profound effects on the person with them. It is not always easy to be cheerful and bright when you have a cold, never mind an unattractive condition that makes you hurt, and to which you can see no end. At least you know that the cold will soon pass; at least you can tell yourself that your spirits will then be restored. People with psoriasis know nothing of the sort.

In most cases of psoriasis the fear of the unknown abates with time. You learn that you can take pleasure from family life, that you can enjoy social occasions, that you can take up new interests and hobbies and that you can be of use to others. And in realizing that the majority of your fears are unfounded, you can get on with your life.

Dealing with negative thinking

Negative thinking often arises from early conditioning. For example, if a woman regularly scoffs at weakness, or if her husband repeatedly declares that incompetence is unforgivable, their children have a fair chance of growing up believing this way of thinking is valid and proper.

When people frequently voice negative thoughts, it generally means they are afraid of the very thing about which they are being negative. The mother who decries weakness does it because she secretly fears she is weak. It is the same with the father who denounces incompetence. His attitude stems from deep-seated doubts about his own competence. When their offspring copy these attitudes into adulthood, condemning weakness and incompetence as well as displaying other negative viewpoints, this, too, stems from the inherent belief that they are lacking in many ways.

Our mindsets – either trust or distrust, enthusiasm or depression, self-assurance or timidity, anxiety or serenity, and so on – usually arise from childhood conditioning. Our automatic thoughts are, therefore, determined by whatever mindsets are built into our character, controlling our behaviour in any given situation. For example, when planning a birthday party, a person with a depressive mindset would dread the 'big day', worrying that few guests would turn up and that he or she hadn't prepared enough food. A person with an enthusiastic mindset, on the other hand, would eagerly await the party, in no doubt at all of its success. A person with a trustful attitude would take the comment, 'That sweater's a bit small for you, love,' as a caring remark and happily change into something that fits better. A person with a distrustful cast of mind, on the other hand, would take it as a criticism of his or her weight, of the sweater, of his or her choice of attire, or of all of these put together!

Irrational feelings

Negative mindsets invariably produce irrational feelings about ourselves – which often become self-fulfilling prophecies. For example, 'I will never be any good with money' stops us trying to be good with money. 'I will never make anyone happy' stops us trying to make anyone happy, and 'I am no fun to have around any more' makes us stop trying to retain a good humour. These irrational feelings are untruths that determine our behaviour. Unfortunately, chronic disease is often the spark that sets irrational feelings blazing out of control.

But these feelings can be turned around. We can learn a new, more positive approach to life. First, however, we need to acknowledge our irrational thoughts and feelings for what they are, and for the behaviour they induce. An upcoming summer barbecue party will commonly provoke feelings of anxiety in a person with psoriasis. Actually writing down your negative thoughts and feelings and really analysing them can make the fact that they are irrational crystal clear. It makes you more aware.

Here is an example of possible irrational thoughts and feelings prior to a summer barbecue party:

Situation	Irrational thoughts	Irrational feelings
Summer barbecue	I can't cover myself from head to toe in this warm weather, so I'll have to put my livid rash on display. Everyone will stare at me in disgust and keep their distance.	I'll feel like a leper and wish I wasn't there.

This example illustrates how irrational a condition such as psoriasis can make a person. Yet without analysis, the potential repercussions can be staggering. In this situation, you may end up talking yourself into staying at home, experiencing mixed self-pity, guilt and even self-loathing. Your decision could even cause an argument with your partner.

The example also reveals a common tendency to worry about something that may never happen. You need, for the sake of sanity, to 'have a life'; you need to be with other people – therefore you need to make an extra effort every now and again. You would feel angry at yourself if you backed out of going to the event, so why not try? Given sufficient forward planning, certain events really can be managed effectively – for whether your symptoms are severe or not, backing out of events and activities that you might have enjoyed can leave you feeling angry at yourself, furious with your condition and resentful that everyone else is 'normal'!

Now try to write down your suppositions about your presence at the barbecue. Look objectively at what you have written. Are your thoughts and feelings reasonable? You probably would feel like a leper if you stood apart from everyone else and made no effort to interact. And could you indeed be so rude as to avoid conversing? Your friends know very well what you look like and the people there whom you don't know – even though they may stare a little at first – will talk and interact with you just as they do everyone else. You know this because they always do, don't they, when you make the effort?

So pick up that pen again and write down your solution to this particular problem.

Situation	Irrational thoughts	Irrational feelings	Solution
Summer barbecue	I can't cover myself from head to toe in this warm weather, so I'll have to put my livid rash on display. Everyone will stare at me in disgust and keep their distance.	I'll feel like a leper and wish I wasn't there.	Wear my best clothes and make a determined effort to join in. Make sure that a good friend stays close by in case I need a little extra help.

When we challenge negative feelings in this way, the reality of the situation soon becomes apparent. People make an effort to be friendly at parties. Your fellow guests are there to enjoy themselves and there will always be someone who wants to chat with you if you're open to that. It's in your hands . . .

Helping others to understand

In attempting to help the people you care about to understand how psoriasis affects you, you should try to speak clearly and openly. Brevity also has a positive impact, as has being honest about how you feel.

Speaking openly

Before trying to describe your feelings, you first need to focus on how you actually do feel. It may be difficult to admit that you feel guilty, frustrated, angry, useless, vulnerable and so on, even to yourself. Sharing your feelings with others is even more difficult, yet it is an important step towards halting the problems that those feelings can cause. In your need to be understood by others, however, you should be wary of making assumptions about how they feel about you.

Speaking to others in the following way is sure to cause offence: 'I know you hate the way I look!' or, 'I don't believe you really care about me, and that makes me feel so hopeless!' or, 'I'm losing confidence because you treat me as if I'm not trying to help myself!' Such comments are likely to be seen as accusations; they may even provoke a quarrel. Speaking directly of your 'emotional problems' – without implying that people you are talking to are contributing to those problems – will encourage them to take your comments more seriously. And it should encourage them to be more thoughtful. Before speaking openly of your feelings, however, do consider the following:

- Ensure that you interpret the other person's behaviour correctly. For example, you may view your mother's bringing you a tub of good moisturizing cream as a criticism of the way you look after yourself, when in truth it is a goodwill gesture, just to show that she cares. You have a perfect right to interpret the words or actions of others in whatever way you wish, but that interpretation is not necessarily reality. In fact, it is amazing how wrong we often are in our perceptions of what others think and feel.

- Ensure that you are specific in recalling another person's behaviour. For example, 'You never understand how embarrassed I get about going out!' is far more inflammatory than 'You didn't seem to understand yesterday, when I told you how embarrassed I felt.'
- Ensure that what you are about to say is what you really mean. For example, statements such as, 'Everyone thinks you're insensitive' or, 'We all think you've got an attitude problem' are, besides being inflammatory, very unfair. We have no way of knowing that 'everyone' is of the same opinion. The use of the depersonalized 'everyone', 'we' or 'us' – often said in the hope of deflecting the listener's anger – can cause far more hurt and anger than if the criticism was direct and personal.

It's easy to see how others can misunderstand or take offence when we fail to communicate effectively. But changing the habits of a lifetime is difficult. It means analysing our thoughts before rearranging them into speech. We are rewarded for our efforts, however, when people start to listen, when they cease to be annoyed as we carefully explain an area they don't fully understood . . . And once we have stopped trying to improve others, we can begin to focus on improving ourselves, and our own situations.

Simplify your life

Being able to focus less on money and material things and more on happiness and fulfilment automatically reduces stress and therefore can improve your psoriasis. Asking yourself the important questions below can help you to re-examine your life and maybe to make changes for the better.

- Do you spend your time idly or otherwise?
- What are the things to which you attach most importance in your life?

- Is your job more stressful than gratifying?
- Could you manage on less money?
- Are you able to say 'no' when you're busy or overextended in some way?
- Are you happy?

Occasional cover-ups

There may be occasional days when you feel particularly self-conscious and would prefer to stay indoors rather than venturing outside. Rather than hiding yourself away, it's always best to go out but cover your psoriasis with clothing or cosmetic cover-up products such as body make-up or a good concealer. Redness and plaques can be masked by such products, but they may irritate the skin and should not be used on cuts, open sores and unhealed lesions.

However, don't, at all costs, get into the habit of covering yourself up. It will only cause numerous self-image problems as well as damage to your self-confidence.

11

Complementary therapies

An increasing number of people with skin conditions are turning to complementary therapies, such as acupuncture, aromatherapy and so on, often in conjunction with their conventional medicines. If you are using or thinking of using complementary therapies, you should be cautious about doing so. Some types can cause adverse reactions and their quality and strength are not controlled by a regulating body. In comparison with mainstream medicine, where a great deal of research has been carried out, there has been very little research and few controlled scientific trials into the effects of complementary medicine. Before deciding to use a particular therapy, try to find out as much about it as you can. You could also ask your doctor's advice. However, the more relaxing therapies can reduce the stress caused by the symptoms of psoriasis.

Acupuncture

An ancient form of Eastern healing, acupuncture involves puncturing the skin with fine needles at specific points in the body. These points are located along energy channels (meridians) that are believed to be blocked where disease is present. This energy is known as chi (also spelt 'qi'). Needles are inserted to increase, decrease or unblock the flow of chi energy so that the balance of yin and yang is restored.

Yin, the female force, is calm and passive; it also represents dark, cold, swelling and moisture. On the other hand, yang, the male force, is stimulating and aggressive, representing heat, light, contraction and dryness. It is thought that an imbalance in these forces is the cause of illness and disease. For example, a person who feels the cold, and suffers fluid retention and fatigue, would be considered to have an excess of yin. A person suffering from repeated headaches, however, will be deemed to have an excess of yang. Emotional, physical or environmental factors are believed to disturb the chi energy balance, and can also be treated. I should mention here that, according to acupuncturists, following a healthy balanced diet, as recommended in Chapter 9, can also go a long way towards restoring the balance of yin and yang.

In your acupuncture session, the therapist determines your particular acupuncture points – it is thought there are as many as 2,000 acupuncture points on the body, and a set method is used to establish where exactly they are. At a consultation, questions may be asked about your lifestyle, sleeping patterns, fears, phobias and reactions to stress. Your pulses will be felt, after which the acupuncture itself is carried out, very fine needles being placed at the relevant sites. The first consultation will normally last for an hour, and you should notice a change for the better after four to six sessions.

Acupuncturists report that they can improve psoriasis by inserting needles along the meridians that correspond to the skin, and also along those that correlate with the underlying causes of the condition. This is said to unblock the energy channels, causing the problem to decline and even to clear completely.

Acupuncture is undoubtedly a very safe therapy. The only very slight risk is that of infection from the needles.

Aromatherapy

Certain health disorders are treated by stimulating our sense of smell with aromatic oils – known as essential oils. Once stimulated, it is believed that a particular smell can help to treat a particular health problem. Indeed, there's no doubt at all that aromatherapy can aid relaxation and help to reduce the anxiety often associated with psoriasis.

Concentrated essential oils are extracted from plants and may be inhaled, rubbed directly into the skin or used in bathing. Each odour relates to its plant of origin – so, for example, lavender oil has the aroma of the lavender plant, and geranium has the aroma of the geranium plant.

Plant essences have been used for healing throughout the ages, smaller amounts being used for aromatherapy purposes than in herbal medicines. Aromatherapy oils are obtained either by steaming a particular plant extract until the oil glands burst, or by soaking the plant extract in hot oil so that the cells collapse and release their essence.

Techniques used in aromatherapy

There are several ways of using aromatherapy. The main ones are:

- Inhalation, which gives the fastest result, since the inhalation of essential oils has a direct influence on the olfactory (nasal) organs, which is immediately received by the brain. Steam inhalation is the most popular technique. This can be achieved either by mixing a few drops of oil with a bowlful of boiling water and leaning over it to breathe in the steam, or by using an oil burner whereby the flame from a tea-light candle heats a small saucer of water containing a few drops of oil.
- Massage, for which the essential oils are normally pre-diluted. They should never be applied to the skin in an undilute (pure) form. When using undiluted essential oils, mix three or four drops with a neutral carrier oil such as olive oil or safflower oil. After penetrating the skin, the oil is absorbed by the body, and the oil is then believed to exert a positive influence on a particular organ or set of tissues. Note that massage oils should not be used on psoriasis plaques or other troublesome or sensitive areas.
- Bathing with oils in the bath water, which can reduce tension and anxiety. A few drops of pure essential oil should be added directly to running tap water – it mixes more efficiently this way. No more than twenty drops of oil in total should be used.

Oils for relaxation

Lavender oil is the most popular oil for relaxation purposes. It is known to be a wonderful restorative and excellent for relieving tension headaches as well as stress. However, there are several others that when used alone or blended can provide a relaxing atmosphere – Roman chamomile and ylang ylang, for example. Ylang ylang has relaxing properties and a calming effect on the heart rate, and it can relieve palpitations and raised blood pressure. Chamomile can be very soothing, too, and aids both sleep and digestion.

Drop your relaxation oils into the vessel part of an oil burner and top up with water. Light a tea-light candle (placed beneath the burner) and try to relax while the essential oils scent the whole room and you inhale their fragrance. Such oils are safe around babies and children, since rather than being overpowering, the aroma is soft and soothing. In recipes 1, 2 and 3, blend the drops well and diffuse them in a burner.

Relaxation recipe 1

5 drops of lavender
2 drops of Roman chamomile
1 drop of ylang ylang

Relaxation recipe 2

8 drops of mandarin
3 drops of neroli
3 drops of ylang ylang

Relaxation recipe 3

10 drops of bergamot
2 drops of rose otto
3 drops of Roman chamomile

Relaxation recipes 2 and 3 can be added to two ounces of distilled water, shaken well and used in a spray bottle for a non-toxic room freshener with relaxing properties.

Relaxation recipe 4

For relaxation, this is a great blend for use in the bath.

3 drops of lavender
2 drops of marjoram
2 drops of basil
1 drop of vetiver
1 drop fennel

Hypnotherapy

Hypnotherapy has been described as psychotherapy using hypnosis. There is, however, still no acceptable definition of the actual state of hypnosis. It is commonly described as an altered state of consciousness, lying somewhere between being awake and being asleep. People under hypnosis are aware of their surroundings, yet their minds are, to a large extent, under the control of the hypnotist. Hypnotized people also seem to pass control of their actions, as well as a chunk of their thoughts, to the hypnotist. We have all seen people under hypnosis on TV, acting out a role. At the time they are absorbed in what they have been 'told' to do – often instigated by a specific 'trigger' word – and immediately afterwards they wonder what on earth they were doing. It's clear that their behaviour had been dictated, to a certain extent, by the hypnotist. Hypno*therapy*, however, is about the hypnotist using the power of hypnotism for therapeutic purposes.

Hypnotherapy is performed by putting the patient into a 'trance' state. You may have heard that, in the early nineteenth century, some surgeons actually used hypnotism – then called 'mesmerism' – to perform pain-free operations. However, the majority of the medical profession at the time were highly sceptical of what these surgeons were doing, believing the patients had been schooled or paid to show no pain. It was not until the last two decades that hypnotism became an accepted form of therapy.

Nowadays, a hypnotherapist will take a full psychological and physiological history of the patient, then slowly talk him or her into a trance state. The therapist can use either direct suggestion – intimating that symptoms will notably lessen – or will begin to explore the root cause of any tension, anxiety or depression. Of course, the exact nature of the therapy depends largely on the problem for which treatment is being sought.

One common fear is that the therapist may, while the patient is in a trance, implant dangerous suggestions, or extract improper personal information. I can only say that patients can come out of a trance at any time – particularly if they are asked to do or say anything that they would not even contemplate when awake. And malpractice would only have to be brought to light once to ruin the therapist's career. You may prefer to visit a hypnotherapist recommended by your doctor.

Some hypnotherapists claim to have had great success in treating psoriasis. They are of the opinion that the condition is a result of repressed emotions, and their aim is to bring such emotions out into the open. Although the main purpose of hypnotherapy is to promote relaxation and reduce tension, it also aims to increase confidence and make a person more able to cope with problems.

There are many anecdotal reports of improvements from using hypnotherapy, but many experts state that there is not enough scientific evidence for them to promote this type of treatment. It is definitely an area worthy of further research, and it is to be hoped this takes place in years to come.

Homoeopathy

The homoeopathic approach to medicine is holistic (i.e. the overall health of a person – physical, emotional and psychological – is assessed before treatment commences). The homoeopathic belief is that the whole make-up of a person determines the disorders to which he or she is prone and the symptoms that are likely to occur. Indeed, homoeopaths profess that their remedies assist the body in its natural tendency to heal itself. A homoeopath will ask you to relate your medical history and personality traits, then offer a remedy compatible with your symptoms as well as with your temperament and characteristics. Consequently, two people with the same disorder may be offered entirely different remedies.

Homoeopathic remedies are derived from plant, mineral and animal substances, which are soaked in alcohol to extract the 'live' ingredients. This initial solution is then diluted many times, being vigorously shaken each time to add energy. Impurities are removed and the remaining solution made up into tablets, ointments, powders or suppositories. Low-dilution remedies are used for severe symptoms while high-dilution remedies are used for milder symptoms.

The homoeopathic concept has, since antiquity, been that 'like cures like'. It is said that the full healing abilities of this type of remedy were first recognized in the early nineteenth century when a German doctor, Samuel Hahnemann, noticed that the herbal cure for malaria – which was based on an extract of cinchona bark (quinine) – actually produced symptoms of malaria. Further tests convinced him that the production of mild symptoms caused the body to fight the disease. He went on to treat malaria patients successfully with dilute doses of cinchona bark.

Each homoeopathic remedy is first 'proved' by being taken by a healthy person – usually a volunteer homoeopath – and the symptoms noted. This remedy is said to be capable of curing the same symptoms in an ill person. The whole idea of 'proving' and using homoeopathic remedies can be difficult to comprehend, since it is exactly the opposite of how conventional medicines operate.

Although the remedies are safe and non-addictive, occasionally the patient's symptoms may worsen briefly. This is known as a healing crisis and is usually short-lived. It is actually a good indication that the remedy is working well.

A range of remedies can be found in most high-street chemists, and more specific ones are available from on-line homoeopathic chemists (see the Useful addresses section at the back of this book for details of one such pharmacy). When self-prescribing, it is advisable to use the 30c potency.

A different homoeopathic approach

Most homoeopaths use conventional remedies for the treatment of psoriasis, as described above. However, some homoeopaths offer a regimen that is tailored specifically for psoriasis. They claim an 80 per cent improvement with some patients, while other patients fail to respond at all.

- Stage 1 involves taking a full case history – this lasts about an hour.
- Stage 2 involves treatment with nutritional supplements, depending upon which are believed to be most suitable. Examples are acidophilus and algae.
- Stage 3 involves a product called neem oil, a rare antiseptic cream from India that is used to soften the skin. You should see results within five sessions.

Biofeedback

Biofeedback is a treatment technique in which people can improve physical and emotional problems by using signals from their own bodies. Physiotherapists use biofeedback to help stroke victims to regain movement in paralysed muscles, and psychologists use it to help anxious clients to learn to relax. Specialists in many different fields use biofeedback to help their patients to cope with pain.

In the late 1960s, when the term 'biofeedback' was first coined, research showed that certain involuntary actions like heart rate, blood pressure and brain function can be altered by tuning into the body. For instance, many people calm anxiety by reading an interesting book. As a result, their heart stops racing and their blood pressure falls to more normal levels. Later research has shown that biofeedback can help in the treatment of many diseases and painful conditions and that we have more control over so-called involuntary function than we once thought possible. Scientists are now trying to determine just how much voluntary control we can exert.

Biofeedback is now widely used to treat pain, high and low blood pressure, paralysis, epilepsy and many other disorders. The technique is taught by psychiatrists, psychologists, doctors and physiotherapists.

A biofeedback specialist will normally teach the following to people with a health problem that is exacerbated by stress:

- a relaxation technique;
- how to identify the circumstances that trigger (or worsen) their symptoms;
- how to cope with events they have previously avoided due to their symptoms;
- how to set attainable goals;
- how to regain control of their life.

In using biofeedback, people must learn to examine their day-to-day life in order to ascertain whether they are somehow contributing to their health problem. They must recognize that they can, by their own efforts, get far more out of their life. In the correct use of biofeedback, bad habits must be changed and, most importantly, the person must accept much of the responsibility for maintaining his or her own health.

Scientists believe that relaxation is the key to the success of this technique. People are taught to react with a calmer frame of mind to certain stimuli – the appearance of an attractive woman or man on a day when they are wearing clothes that reveal the psoriasis, for instance. As a result, the stress response is not triggered and adrenalin is not pumped into the bloodstream. Without biofeedback training, adrenalin may be released repeatedly, causing chronic anxiety, stress, muscle tension and depression.

If you think you might benefit from biofeedback training, you should discuss the matter with your doctor.

Reflexology

Reflexology, an ancient Eastern therapy, was only recently adopted in the Western world. It operates on the proposition that the body is divided into different energy zones, all of which can be exploited in the prevention and treatment of any disorder.

Reflexologists have identified ten energy channels beginning in the toes and extending to the fingers and top of the head. Each channel relates to a particular bodily zone, and to the organs in that zone. For example, the big toe relates to the head (the brain, ears, sinus area, neck, pituitary glands and eyes). By applying pressure to the appropriate terminal in the form of a small, specialized massage, a practitioner can determine which energy pathways are blocked.

Experts in this type of manipulative therapy claim that all the organs of the body are reflected in the feet. They also believe that reflexology aids the removal of waste products and blockages within the energy channels, improving circulation and lymph gland function. Reflexology is certainly relaxing – for the mind and body. Indeed, as well as reducing stress, it can improve depression.

Many therapists prefer to take down a full case history before commencing treatment. Each session will take up to 45 minutes (the preliminary session may take longer), and you will be treated sitting in a chair or lying down.

Relaxation

Long-term frustration and anxiety invariably lead to chronic stress – the state of being constantly 'on alert'. The physiological changes associated with this state – a fast heart rate, shallow breathing and muscular tension – often persist over a long period, making relaxation very difficult. Chronic stress can lead to nerviness, hypertension, irritability and depression.

Deep breathing

In normal breathing, we take oxygen from the atmosphere down into our lungs. The diaphragm contracts and air is pulled into the chest cavity. When we breathe out, we expel carbon dioxide and other waste gases back into the atmosphere. But when we are stressed or upset, we tend to use the rib muscles to expand the chest. We breathe more quickly, sucking in shallowly. This is excellent in a crisis because it allows us to obtain the optimum amount of oxygen in the shortest possible time, providing our bodies with the extra power needed to handle the emergency. Some people do tend to get stuck in chest-breathing mode, however. Long-term shallow breathing is not only detrimental to physical and emotional health, it can also lead to hyperventilation, panic attacks, chest pains, dizziness and gastrointestinal problems.

To test your breathing, ask yourself:

- How fast are you breathing as you are reading this?
- Are you pausing between breaths?
- Are you breathing with your chest or with your diaphragm?

A breathing exercise

The following deep breathing exercise should, ideally, be performed daily.

1 Ensure that you are not wearing tight clothing. If you are, change into something loose-fitting.
2 Make yourself comfortable in a warm room where you know you will be alone for at least half an hour.
3 Close your eyes and try to relax.
4 Gradually slow down your breathing, inhaling and exhaling as evenly as possible.

5 Place one hand on your chest and the other on your abdomen, just below your rib-cage.

6 As you inhale, allow your abdomen to swell upward. (Your chest should barely move.)

7 As you exhale, let your abdomen flatten.

Give yourself a few minutes to get into a smooth, easy rhythm. As worries and distractions arise, don't hang on to them. Wait calmly for them to float out of your mind – then focus once more on your breathing.

When you feel ready to end the exercise, open your eyes. Allow yourself time to become alert before getting up. With practice, you will begin breathing with your diaphragm quite naturally – and in times of stress, you should be able to correct your breathing without too much effort.

Stress-busting suggestions

If your psoriasis makes you feel stressed in any way, try to put into practice the stress-busting suggestions below. Carrying out at least two or three different ones every day should enable you to cope better with your day-to-day life.

- Smile as often as you can.
- Drive in the slow lane.
- Perform your daily activities at a slower pace – walking, eating, reading, doing the housework, washing the car, doing the cross-word puzzle and so on.
- Stop yourself from grimacing.
- Buy a small gift for someone you care about.
- Tell someone you care about how much they mean to you.
- Pay someone a compliment.
- Refer to yourself less frequently in conversation.
- Practise controlling your anger.
- Allow yourself to cry if you feel like doing so.
- Practise assertiveness.
- Listen to music.
- Take a long bath.
- Alter your routine slightly.
- Take a leisurely walk around a park or through woodland.
- Notice nature more – flowers, birds, trees, rainbows and sunsets.

A relaxation exercise

Relaxation is one of the forgotten skills in today's hectic world. However, learning at least one relaxation technique can counter the stress arising from psoriasis symptoms and anxiety over its appearance. The following exercise is perhaps the easiest.

1 Ensure that you are not wearing tight clothing.
2 Make yourself comfortable in a place where you will not be disturbed. (Listening to restful music may help you relax.)
3 Begin to slow down your breathing, inhaling through your nose to a count of two.
4 Exhale to a count of four, five or six, ensuring that the abdomen swells upwards as air leaves your mouth . . .
5 After a couple of minutes, concentrate on each part of your body in turn, starting with your right arm. Consciously relax each set of muscles, allowing the tension to flow right out . . . Let your arm feel heavier and heavier as every last remnant of tension seeps away . . . Follow this procedure with the muscles of your left arm, then the muscles of your face, your neck, your stomach, your hips and finally your legs.

Visualization

At this point, visualization can be introduced into the exercise. As you continue to breathe slowly and evenly, imagine yourself surrounded, perhaps, by lush, peaceful countryside, beside a gently trickling stream – or maybe on a deserted tropical beach, beneath swaying palm fronds, listening to the sounds of the ocean, thousands of miles from your worries and cares. Let the warm sun, the gentle breeze, the peacefulness of it all wash over you.

The tranquillity you feel at this stage can be enhanced by repeating the exercise frequently – once or twice a day is best. With time, you should be able to switch into a calm state of mind whenever you feel stressed.

Meditation

Arguably the oldest natural therapy, meditation is the simplest and most effective form of self-help. Dr Herbert Benson of Harvard Medical School has been able to show that meditation tends to normalize blood pressure, pulse rate and the level of stress hormones in the blood. He has proved, too, that it produces changes in brain wave patterns (showing less excitability) and that it strengthens the immune system and endocrine system (which produces the body's hormones).

The unusual thing about meditation is that it involves 'letting go', allowing the mind to roam freely. Most of us are used to trying to control our thoughts – in our work, for example – and therefore letting go is not as easy as it sounds.

It may help to know that people who regularly meditate say they have more energy, require less sleep, are less anxious and feel far 'more alive' than before they did so. Ideally, the technique should be taught by a teacher – but, since meditation is essentially performed alone, it can be learned alone with equal success.

Meditation may, to some people, sound a bit off-beat. But isn't it worth a try? Especially when you can do it for free! Kick off those shoes and make yourself comfortable, somewhere you can be alone for a while. Now follow these simple instructions:

1 Close your eyes, relax, and practise the deep breathing exercise as described above.
2 Concentrate on your breathing. Try to free your mind of conscious control.
3 Letting your mind roam unchecked, try to allow the deeper, more serene part of you to take over.
4 If you wish to go further into meditation, concentrate on mentally repeating a mantra – a certain word or phrase. It should be something positive, such as 'relax', 'I feel calm' or even 'I am special'.
5 When you are ready to finish, open your eyes and allow yourself time to adjust to the outside world before getting to your feet.

The aim of repeating a mantra is to plant positive thoughts into your subconscious mind. It is a form of self-hypnosis, and you alone control the messages placed there.

Useful addresses

Organizations concerned specifically with psoriasis

UK

The Psoriasis Association
Dick Coles House
2 Queensbridge
Northampton NN4 7BF
Tel.: 0845 676 0076/01604 251620
Website: www.psoriasis-association.org.uk

This association is the leading national membership-based organization for people affected by psoriasis – patients, families, carers and health professionals. Its aims are to support people with psoriasis, to raise awareness and to fund research into the causes, treatments and care of the condition. There is a quarterly journal for members.

The Psoriasis and Psoriatic Arthritis Alliance (formerly the Psoriatic Arthropathy Alliance)
PO Box 111
St Albans
Herts AL2 3JQ
Tel.: 0870 770 3212
Website: www.papaa.org

The Alliance was founded in 2007 as a joint venture between the Psoriatic Arthropathy Alliance and the Psoriasis Support Trust. Run by patients for patients, this group produces a helpful newsletter and organizes an annual conference.

Overseas

National Psoriasis Foundation
6600 SW 92nd Avenue, Suite 300
Portland
Oregon 97223-7195
USA
Tel.: (800) 723 9166
Website: www.psoriasis.org

This US foundation is the world's largest non-profit organization dedicated to educating, serving and empowering people with psoriasis and psoriatic arthritis.

Psoriasis Association of New Zealand Inc.
PO Box 44007
Lower Hutt
Wellington 6315
New Zealand
Tel.: (04) 568 7139
Website: www.everybody.co.nz

This membership-based association in New Zealand aims to educate those with psoriasis about the condition and about available treatments. It also seeks to raise public awareness, encourages research, distributes information and provides social interaction for its members.

Psoriasis Australia
PO Box 290
Ashburton
Victoria 3147
Australia
Tel.: (03) 9813 8080
Website: www.psoriasisaustralia.
org.au

This Australian association aims to
help people with psoriasis and their
families by providing information
and support. It holds quarterly
meetings that feature guest
speakers, and there is a quarterly
newsletter.

Psoriasis Society of Canada
PO Box 25015
Halifax
Nova Scotia B3M 4H4
Canada
Tel.: (902) 443 8680
Website: www.psoriasissociety.org

This Canadian organization gives
details of local support groups,
helps to raise public awareness and
encourages research into psoriasis.

General

UK

**The British Association of
Dermatologists**
Willan House
4 Fitzroy Square
London W1T 5HQ
Tel.: 020 7383 0266
Website: www.bad.org.uk

This is the central association of
practising UK dermatologists. Its
aim is to improve continually
the treatment and understanding

of skin disease by raising public
awareness and supporting its
members.

British Nutrition Foundation
High Holborn House
52–54 High Holborn
London WC1V 6RQ
Tel.: 020 7404 6504
Website: www.nutrition.org.uk

This website provides healthy
eating information, resources for
schools, news items, recipes and
details of the work the Foundation
undertakes around the UK and in
the rest of the EU.

Disability Alliance
Universal House
88–94 Wentworth Street
London E1 7SA
Tel.: 020 7247 8776 (voice and
minicom)
Website: www.disabilityalliance.org

This is a charitable organization,
which publishes the *Disability
Rights Handbook*. Its aim is to
improve the living standards of
disabled people by breaking the
link between poverty and disability.
It achieves this by providing a
variety of services to disabled
people, their families, carers and
professional advisers, through
advice, information, campaign
work, research and training.

Pure Skin Care
Tel.: 0121 288 3962
Website: www.pureskincare.co.uk

This is an internet-based shop
selling a range of skincare products
made with organic and natural
ingredients.

USA

American Academy of Dermatology
PO Box 4014
Schaumburg
Illinois 60618-4014
USA
Tel.: (847) 330 0230
Website: www.aad.org

The American Academy of Dermatology is the largest, most influential and most representative of all membership-based dermatological associations. The Academy is committed to excellence in patient care, medical and public education, research, professionalism and member service and support. There is no email contact.

National Institute of Arthritis and Musculoskeletal and Skin Diseases
Information Clearinghouse
National Institutes of Health
1 AMS Circle
Bethesda
Maryland 20892-3675
USA
Tel.: (301) 495 4484
Website: www.niams.nih.gov

This US 'clearinghouse' serves the public, patients and health professionals by providing information, locating other information sources, creating health education materials and participating in a national database on health topics.

References

1 Williams, R. C., McKenzie, A. W., Roger, J. H. and Joysey, V. C., 'HL-A antigens in patients with guttate psoriasis'. *British Journal of Dermatology*, vol. 95, pp. 163–7, 1976.

2 Picardi, A. and Abeni, D., 'Stressful life events and skin diseases: disentangling evidence from myth'. *Journal of Psychotherapy and Psychosomatics*, vol. 70, pp. 118–36, 2001.

3 Al-Suwaidan, S. N. and Feldman, S. R., 'Clearance is not a realistic goal of psoriasis treatment'. *Journal of the American Academy of Dermatology*, vol. 42, pp. 796–802, 2000.

4 Christophers, E., Mrowietz, U., Henneicke, H. H., Färber, L. and Welzel, D., 'Cyclosporine in psoriasis: a multicenter dose-finding study in severe plaque psoriasis'. *Journal of the American Academy of Dermatology*, vol. 26, pp. 86–90, 1992.

5 Goldfarb, M. T., Ellis, C. N., Gupta, A. K., Tincoff, T., Hamilton T. A. and Voorhees, J. J., 'Acitretin improves psoriasis in a dose dependent fashion'. *Journal of the American Academy of Dermatology*, vol. 18, pp. 655–62, 1988.

6 Berbis, P., Geiger, J. M., Vaisse, C., Rognin, C. and Privat, Y., 'Benefit of progressively increasing doses during the initial treatment with acitretin in psoriasis'. *Dermatologica*, vol. 178, pp. 88–92, 1989.

7 Stern, R. S. and Laird, N., 'The carcinogenic risk of treatments for severe psoriasis. Photochemotherapy follow-up study'. *Cancer*, vol. 73, pp. 2759–64, 1994.

8 Stern, R. S., Nichols, K. T. and Väkevä, L. H., 'Malignant melanoma in patients treated for psoriasis with methoxsalen (psoralen) and ultraviolet A radiation (PUVA)'. *New England Journal of Medicine*, vol. 336, pp. 1041–5, 1997.

Further reading

Camisa, Charles, *Handbook of Psoriasis*. WileyBlackwell, Malden, Massachusetts, USA, 2005.

Creagan, Edward T. and Mayo Clinic, *Mayo Clinic Book of Alternative Medicine: Making Alternative Therapies Part of Your Healthy Lifestyle*. Time Inc. Home Entertainment, New York, 2007.

Earls, Deidre, *Your Healing Diet: A Quick Guide to Reversing Psoriasis and Chronic Diseases with Healing Foods*. Booksurge, North Charleston, South Carolina, USA, 2005.

Lewis, Jenny, *The Psoriasis Handbook: A Definitive Guide to the Causes, Symptoms and All the Latest Treatments*. Vermilion, London, 1996.

Lowe, N. J., *Psoriasis: A Patient's Guide*. Taylor and Francis, London, 2003.

Mitchell, Tim and Penzer, Rebecca, *Psoriasis: The At Your Fingertips Guide*. Class Publishing, London, 2005.

Schwartz, Mark S. and Andrasik, Frank, *Biofeedback: A Practitioner's Guide*. Guilford Publications, New York, 2005.

Warin, Andrew, *Understanding Psoriasis*. Family Doctor Publications, Poole, 2005.

Index

alcohol 47, 64, 99–100
arthritis mutilans 22
artificial nails 31
autoimmune antibodies 44–5

blood vessels 14–15
body temperature 12–16

cell division 4
children (with psoriasis) 6, 24, 36, 107
climate 3, 16
complementary therapies 116–28
  acupuncture 116–17
  aromatherapy 117–19
  biofeedback 123–4
  homoeopathy 121–2
  hypnotherapy 120–1
  reflexology 124
confidence 104
corticosteroids, topical 52–5
cosmetic hair treatments 32–3

Dead Sea 56
diagnosis 20–3

eczema 16–17
emotional help 103–15
  helping others to understand 113–14
  irrational feelings 111–13
  negative emotions 108
  negative thinking 110
  simplify your life 114–15
exercise 84–5

flare-up 29–30, 32, 37, 45–6
forms of psoriasis
  erythrodermic 41–2
  guttate 35–9
  inverse 39–41
  nail 26–31
  plaque 9–17
  psoriatic arthritis 19–26

pustular 2–4
scalp 31–5

genetics
  CDSN gene 43–4

herbal remedies 88
HIV (human immunodeficiency virus) 20, 46, 48

immune system 1, 19, 23, 46, 48, 128
  B cells 44–5
  leukocytes 44
  lymphocytes 44
  mast cells 39
  T cells 44, 72, 90
  TH cells 44–5
infection 46
inflammation 9, 15, 19–23, 25, 53
injections 61–74
intimacy 106
itching 10, 31, 38, 41, 51, 103, 106

lesions 6, 12, 29, 32, 34–6, 39–41

medicated shampoos 35
medications 25–6, 47–9, 64
  acitretin 65
  biologic response modifiers 71–4
  ciclosporin 67–8
  corticosteroids 34
  folic acid 63–4
  hydroxyurea (hydroxycarbamide) 70–1
  isotretinoin 66–7
  methotrexate 25, 62–3
  oral retinoids 65
  sulfasalazine 69–70

nutrition 92–102

obesity 46
occlusive dressings 59–60
oestrogen 7

phototherapy 75–9
  broadband UVB 77–8
  laser treatment 78
  narrowband UVB 78
  PUVA therapy 76–7
pregnancy 6–7, 54, 64

rash 2, 5, 9, 36–7, 47
relaxation 125–8
  meditation 127–8
  visualization 127
retinoids, topical 57–8

seborrhoeic dermatitis 33
self-help 80
skin cancer 4, 51, 68–9, 75–6, 81
skin function 15
  dermis 13
  epidermis 13
  keratinization 13
  keratinocytes 14–15
smoking 47, 82, 100

spondylitis 20
streptococcal infection 36–9
streptococcus bacterium 37
stress 104, 108, 114, 126–27
sunlight 64
surgery 26
systemic agents 49

tanning beds 78
topical treatments 49–60
  anthralin 55–6
  coal tar 33, 51–2
  corticosteroids 52–5
  emollients 50–1
  moisturizers 51
  retinoids 57–8
  salicylic acid 58
Trembath, Richard 43–4
triggering factors 46

vitamin D compounds 56
vaccine 24